Behind The Filtered Smiles

Prologue

In the age of digital masks, where authenticity was a scarce commodity, Kieran sat in his dimly lit bedroom, scrolling through his Instagram feed. He watched as his finger swiped past perfectly curated images, each one a carefully constructed facade of happiness, success, and charm. The lives of his friends and acquaintances unfolded before him in an endless stream of snapshots and stories, all wrapped in a shimmering veneer of edited perfection.

He sighed, his own insecurities bubbling up like a dormant volcano. Kieran was no stranger to the art of social media deception. In his virtual world, he was a dazzling star, a portrait of unblemished confidence and boundless charisma. But in reality, he was a twenty-something introvert, his self-esteem hanging by the thinnest of threads.

"Kieran, you're an influencer," his friends would often remind him, amused by the stark contrast between his online persona and his offline self. He had thousands of followers who admired his glamorous lifestyle, but the applause and adoration were built on a foundation of artifice. The deeper he dove into this digital masquerade, the harder it became to extricate himself from its web of lies.

Tonight, as Kieran stared at his phone, he felt a growing sense of disillusionment. He knew that he was far from alone in this world of make-believe. The entire internet was a theater, a stage for people to perform as characters they wished they could be in reality. He had once believed he could juggle both his true self and his fabricated online persona, but the lines had blurred, and he no longer knew where one ended and the other began.

He glanced at his reflection in the mirror, pondering the guy with the perfectly styled hair, flawless beard, and impeccable outfits that his followers adored. His gaze lingered on his own eyes, a shade of blue that had lost its luster. There, beneath the mask, he saw a flicker of sadness and longing.

As the hours slipped away, Kieran couldn't help but wonder: Who was he, really? Did he even know himself anymore? And could he ever escape the clutches of the digital puppeteer he had become?

In this book, we'll delve into the life of Kieran, who walks the tightrope between reality and illusion, exploring the complexities of a world where everyone portrays a fake persona on social media, and the profound impact it has on their lives.

The dark road that "KaiZen" led Kieran down, exploring the toll it takes on his mental health and the fragile line he walks between the digital persona he had created and the real person he once was. The journey will be a poignant exploration of the highs and lows of living in the age of social media, a world where the pursuit of perfection can lead to a harrowing descent into the depths of one's own psyche.

Chapter 1
Behind The Filtered Smiles

Kieran possessed a striking, enigmatic presence that drew attention wherever he went. His tall, athletic frame exuded an air of confidence, and his impeccable style made him stand out in any crowd. People couldn't help but notice his chiseled jawline and piercing blue eyes that seemed to hold a universe of unspoken stories.

However, upon closer examination, one would discern the subtle imperfections that added depth and character to his appearance. Kieran bore the remnants of a battle with teenage acne, with a constellation of faint but visible scars scattered across his cheeks and forehead. These scars, though once a source of self-consciousness, now told a story of resilience and personal growth.

One scar, in particular, drew curious glances from those who were fortunate enough to catch a glimpse of his bare chest. It was a long, silvery line etched across his pectoral muscle, a testament to a traumatic incident from his past. Kieran rarely spoke about it, but the scar served as a reminder of a challenge he had faced and conquered.

His face, framed by a well-maintained beard that accentuated his strong jawline, had a rugged charm that made him approachable and relatable. His eyes, the shade of a deep, endless sea, held a certain vulnerability that contradicted his confident demeanor. They were windows to a soul that had weathered storms and found strength in the midst of adversity.

Kieran's physique was a testament to his dedication to fitness. He had honed his body through years of disciplined workouts and a commitment to a healthy lifestyle. Muscles rippled beneath his skin, defined by hours of strenuous exercise, and he moved with a fluid grace that commanded attention without demanding it.

Yet, beneath the allure of his appearance lay a complex tapestry of emotions. The acne scars on his face, though faded, carried with them the echoes of a time when he had battled insecurity and self-doubt. The chest scar told a story of pain and recovery, a reminder that strength could emerge from vulnerability.

Kieran's outer beauty was not a facade to mask deeper issues; instead, it was a reflection of his journey towards self-acceptance. It was a testament to his capacity to embrace imperfections and use them to build a resilient and captivating personality.

Kieran's dual existence starts to unfold, these physical imperfections serve as metaphors for the inner struggles he faces, hinting at the complexities of his character and the mental health issues that lurk beneath the surface. His journey is not just about maintaining a dual persona on social media but also about confronting and healing the scars that life has left on his body and soul.

Kieran's obsession with the world of social media influencers and their seemingly flawless lives was a daily ritual. As he sat alone in his dimly lit bedroom, scrolling through his Instagram feed, he couldn't help but marvel at the carefully cultivated images of these digital idols. The sheer perfection of their online personas was both a source of admiration and envy.

For Kieran, the perfect skin that adorned the faces of these digital gods was like a siren's call, a reminder of the imperfections that marred his own complexion. He often found himself fixated on images of influencers with flawless, airbrushed skin. Their faces were untouched by the scars of acne or the blemishes that Kieran had learned to accept as part of his own story. These idols seemed to possess an otherworldly beauty that he longed for, an unattainable standard that fueled his obsession.

In addition to their perfect skin, these influencers flaunted bodies that seemed sculpted by the gods themselves. Their photographs were a celebration of chiseled abs, toned muscles, and graceful curves. Kieran's physique was the result of hard work and dedication, but when compared to the seemingly effortless perfection of his idols, he couldn't help but feel inadequate. He yearned to possess the same flawless physique that adorned their social media profiles, longing to be free of the insecurities that gnawed at him from within.

Trinkets of expensive possessions, gleaming in meticulously posed photographs, were another facet of this digital utopia. Kieran was entranced by the way his idols effortlessly showcased luxury cars, designer clothing, and exotic vacations. The images of their opulent lives were a stark contrast to his own modest reality. He had often wondered what it would be like to live without financial constraints, to own the coveted possessions that seemed to define success in the world of social media.

But it wasn't just the material possessions that captivated Kieran. It was the aura of glamour and opulence that surrounded these influencers. Their lives appeared to be an unending celebration of luxury, a relentless pursuit of the extravagant. Kieran couldn't help but feel a sense of longing as he scrolled through their images, wondering what it would be like to live in a world of boundless abundance.

Perfect photos were the final element of this digital wonderland that Kieran revered. The artful compositions, impeccable lighting, and flawless editing left him in awe. The images were more than just photographs; they were carefully crafted masterpieces that showcased the influencers in their best light. Kieran often compared these pictures to the candid, unfiltered snapshots he took of himself, and the disparity left him feeling inadequate.

The idolatry of these social media figures was more than just an innocent admiration; it was a deep-seated yearning to escape the imperfections of his own life. Their lives, as portrayed on Instagram, seemed to be the epitome of happiness, success, and beauty. Kieran couldn't help but think that if he could achieve just a fraction of what these idols had, he would be content.

The obsession with these perfect digital idols served as both motivation and torment for Kieran. On one hand, it inspired him to improve himself, to work on his physique and appearance, and to strive for success. But on the other hand, it also fueled his anxiety and self-doubt. The unattainable standards he held himself to left him in a constant state of unease, as if he were chasing an ever-elusive dream.

In this digital world of curated perfection, Kieran's mental health was at stake. The relentless comparison to these idols, each with their unblemished skin, idealized bodies, expensive possessions, and flawless photos, left him teetering on the precipice of self-destruction. The quest for an unattainable ideal was slowly eroding his sense of self-worth, and he was about to confront a deeper truth – that the images he worshipped were as much a façade as his own dual persona on social media.

In the early days of his social media journey, Kieran was just like any other user. His profile was a collection of random posts, snapshots of everyday life, and occasional selfies taken with little thought. It was a reflection of his authentic self, a canvas that revealed his unfiltered, unedited existence. But as Kieran delved deeper into the world of digital influencers, he realized that authenticity alone wouldn't help him gain the coveted following he desired.

He had seen countless influencers who had managed to craft a persona so alluring, so magnetic, that it drew followers in like moths to a flame. These influencers had a knack for presenting a perfect, curated image, an image that Kieran couldn't help but envy. It was as if they had unlocked the secret to a world of boundless admiration and affirmation.

Kieran began to analyze their profiles meticulously, studying every detail, every post, and every caption. He noticed a pattern, a carefully orchestrated symphony of elements that made up the enchanting personas of these digital stars. They had a color scheme that was consistent throughout their feed, creating a sense of harmony and cohesion. Kieran observed how they used specific filters and photo editing techniques to enhance their images, making them radiate an ethereal glow. It was as if they had a personal brand, a unique signature that set them apart in the crowded digital landscape.

But it wasn't just the visual aspect that caught Kieran's attention. The captions were equally important. He noticed that his idols had a way with words, crafting captions that were both relatable and aspirational. Their words were carefully chosen to invoke a sense of connection with their followers, to make them feel seen and understood. Kieran realized that the art of storytelling was a powerful tool in their arsenal. These influencers could take the most mundane aspects of their lives and spin them into tales of inspiration and motivation.

Kieran was determined to emulate this formula for success. He knew that if he wanted to gain followers and become accepted in the flawless world of digital social media, he had to transform his profile into something that was both visually appealing and emotionally engaging.

The transformation began with the curation of his feed. Kieran selected a color palette that resonated with his personal style, settling on a combination of cool blues and warm earth tones. He meticulously organized his posts to create a sense of harmony, ensuring that no clashing colors disrupted the visual flow of his feed. It was a tedious process, but he was willing to put in the effort to achieve the desired aesthetic.

Photo editing became his new obsession. Kieran experimented with various filters and editing apps, learning how to enhance the lighting, contrast, and saturation of his images. He found himself spending hours perfecting each photo, erasing blemishes and imperfections, and creating a soft, dreamy glow that mimicked the look of his idols. Every image was a labor of love, a digital masterpiece that he hoped would capture the attention of potential followers.

The art of storytelling was the next mountain to conquer. Kieran began to pay closer attention to the narratives that accompanied his idols' posts. He realized that they were masters of vulnerability, opening up about their insecurities, their struggles, and their triumphs. It was a delicate balance of authenticity and aspiration. Kieran decided to share more of his personal journey, to reveal the challenges he had faced and the goals he aspired to achieve. It was a way to connect with his audience on a deeper level, to let them know that he was just like them, striving for success and self-improvement.

Kieran's profile began to evolve, and with it, so did his online persona. He was no longer just an observer; he had become a participant in the world of digital influencers. His posts exuded a newfound confidence and charisma, as if he had tapped into a wellspring of self-assuredness. His followers began to notice the change, and the likes and comments started pouring in. Kieran was gaining the attention and affirmation he had longed for.

But as his digital alter ego flourished, a subtle transformation was occurring within him. The line between his authentic self and his online persona was blurring, and he found himself living a dual existence. Kieran relished in the attention and admiration, but he also began to feel the weight of the expectations he had set for himself. The flawless world of digital social media was a double-edged sword, and Kieran was about to discover the toll it would take on his mental and emotional well-being.

Kieran knew that to truly immerse himself in the world of digital influencers, he needed a name, an identity that would resonate with his future followers. After careful consideration, he decided on the moniker "KaiZen." The name was a fusion of two concepts: "Kai," representing change and transformation, and "Zen," symbolizing balance and harmony. It was a reflection of his desire for personal growth and a life in equilibrium, a name that held a promise of continual self-improvement.

As "KaiZen," he would present himself as a beacon of positivity, a testament to the power of change and self-evolution. He believed that the name encapsulated his journey and his aspiration to balance the imperfections of his real life with the polished perfection of his online presence. It was a name that embodied his hope for continuous improvement and his commitment to inspiring others to follow a similar path.

The transformation into "KaiZen" was complete. He had created a visually appealing profile, honed his photo-editing skills, and mastered the art of storytelling. Now, he had a name that would become synonymous with his digital alter ego, a name that he hoped would draw followers into his world of curated perfection.

As "KaiZen," he began posting with a newfound enthusiasm, sharing the most inspiring aspects of his life. Each post was an opportunity to showcase his commitment to change and self-improvement. The captions were laced with motivation, encouraging his followers to embrace their imperfections and embark on their own journeys of transformation. It was as if "KaiZen" had become a digital mentor, guiding his followers toward a life of balance and harmony.

But as "KaiZen" continued to rise in popularity, Kieran found himself grappling with the dual nature of his existence. The persona of "KaiZen" was a polished image of success, but the real Kieran was still plagued by insecurities and doubts. The flawless world of digital social media was both a refuge and a prison, a place where he had created a persona that was adored and admired, yet one that was slowly eroding his sense of self.

As the story unfolds, Kieran's struggle with maintaining his "KaiZen" persona while reconciling it with his authentic self becomes a central theme. The name "KaiZen" represents not just his online identity, but also the aspiration for personal growth and the delicate balance he seeks to achieve between the digital world and reality. Kieran will grapple with the complexities of living a dual existence and the toll it takes on his mental and emotional well-being, a poignant journey that delves deep into the intricacies of the human psyche in the age of social media.

Little did Kieran know what "KaiZen" would become and the dark road that lay ahead. At first, his digital alter ego had been a source of inspiration, a symbol of hope and personal growth. But as "KaiZen" gained followers and the pressure to maintain the facade grew, Kieran found himself slipping down a treacherous path.

The perfection he portrayed on social media began to consume him. "KaiZen" was no longer a reflection of his authentic self but an idealized version that he could barely recognize. The relentless pursuit of curated perfection had transformed him into a prisoner of his own creation.

Kieran, the real person behind the screen, had taken a back seat to "KaiZen." He found it increasingly challenging to differentiate between the two personas. The line between his digital alter ego and his true self had blurred to the point of non-existence. It was a dichotomy that tormented him, a constant struggle to reconcile the flawless world of "KaiZen" with the imperfections of Kieran.

As he continued down this dark road, Kieran began to feel the weight of the expectations he had set for himself. The pressure to maintain the illusion of boundless success and happiness was suffocating. His obsession with gaining followers and keeping up appearances left him in a state of perpetual anxiety. The real Kieran, the introverted young man with acne scars and a chest scar, was drowning beneath the polished veneer of "KaiZen."

The digital utopia he had longed to be a part of was now a digital dystopia, a place where his mental health crumbled under the relentless pressure to conform to the standards he had created. The flawless world of digital social media was no longer a refuge; it had become a prison, a place where Kieran was a captive of his own creation.

In his journey, Kieran would confront the dark side of the digital world, a side that was often obscured by the façade of curated perfection. The story would delve into the profound impact of social media on mental health, exploring the toll it took on Kieran's psyche as he grappled with his dual existence and the relentless quest for likes, followers, and validation.

Chapter 2
Digital Sirens

As Kieran delved deeper into the world of social media influencers, he found himself increasingly captivated by the allure of illusion. Each post, each carefully crafted image, was a siren's call, beckoning him further into a world where reality and aspiration danced in perfect harmony.

He spent hours studying the profiles of his digital idols, dissecting their posts like a scientist examining a complex equation. It wasn't just about the images; it was about the stories they told, the emotions they evoked, and the dreams they inspired. Kieran realized that these influencers were not just curators of content; they were masters of storytelling, weaving narratives that transported their followers to distant lands, glamorous events, and a life filled with endless adventure.

One day, as he scrolled through the profile of "SoleilWanderlust," he stumbled upon a post that struck a chord deep within him. It was a photograph of her standing on the edge of a cliff, her arms outstretched, as if she were about to take flight. The backdrop was a breathtaking vista of rolling hills and a cerulean sky, a scene straight out of a fantasy novel.

The caption read, "Leap of faith into the unknown. □ Sometimes, all it takes is a single moment of courage to change your life forever. #AdventureAwaits #FearlessDreamer #Limitless."

Kieran couldn't help but be moved by those words. They resonated with a part of him that had longed for something more, something beyond the confines of his everyday existence. The photograph was a symbol of freedom, of breaking free from the constraints of fear and doubt. It was a testament to the power of taking risks and embracing the unknown.

Inspired by the allure of SoleilWanderlust's post, Kieran decided to take a leap of faith of his own. He wanted to be more than just an observer; he wanted to be a participant in this world of digital sorcery. He was determined to craft a persona that would captivate and inspire, just like his idols had done for him.

The transformation began with a series of carefully curated posts. Kieran embarked on a journey of self-discovery, seeking out experiences that would not only enrich his life but also provide fodder for his digital alter ego. He traveled to exotic locations, dined at fashionable restaurants, and attended glamorous events, all the while documenting his adventures with expertly crafted photographs and captions.

Each post was a performance, a carefully orchestrated act that presented "KaiZen" as a fearless dreamer, a seeker of adventure, and a master of self-improvement. Kieran learned the art of posing, the magic of lighting, and the secrets of photo editing. He spent countless hours perfecting his craft, obsessively chasing the elusive illusion of perfection.

As "KaiZen," Kieran's profile began to transform into a digital dreamscape. His followers grew in number, and his posts garnered more likes and comments with each passing day. He had become a digital sorcerer in his own right, wielding the power of illusion to captivate his audience.

But as the digital sirens lured him further into their world of enchantment, Kieran couldn't help but wonder about the toll this pursuit was taking on his authentic self. The line between "KaiZen" and Kieran was becoming increasingly blurred, and he found himself living a dual existence.

Kieran's desire to create a better version of himself was a driving force behind his transformation into "KaiZen." He had always harbored aspirations for self-improvement, but in the world of social media, those aspirations took on a new dimension. He saw the opportunity to not only become a better version of himself but also to present that version to the world, to showcase a life of endless growth and potential.

As "KaiZen," he felt liberated from the constraints of his own insecurities and doubts. He could shed the imperfections that had weighed him down and step into a world where he was the master of his own destiny. It was a world where he could chase dreams without fear, where he could embrace challenges with unwavering confidence, and where he could become the person he had always wanted to be.

Kieran's posts were a testament to this pursuit of self-improvement. He shared his journey of self-discovery, documenting the books he read, the skills he learned, and the personal milestones he achieved. He presented "KaiZen" as a relentless seeker of knowledge and a fearless explorer of life's possibilities. It was as if he had unlocked the secret to continual growth, and he wanted to inspire others to follow a similar path.

The desire to create a better version of himself was not just about personal fulfillment; it was also about the impact he could have on his followers. Kieran wanted to be a source of inspiration and motivation, a digital mentor who could guide others toward a life of balance and harmony. He believed that by showcasing his own journey of self-improvement, he could empower others to embark on their own quests for personal growth.

But as Kieran continued on this path, he couldn't help but question the authenticity of his pursuit. Was he truly becoming a better version of himself, or was he simply creating a polished illusion of improvement? The line between reality and aspiration was becoming increasingly blurred, and Kieran was about to confront the consequences of his relentless pursuit of perfection.

What Kieran admired most about digital influencers was their ability to craft a world of inspiration and aspiration. As he immersed himself further into the digital realm, he found himself increasingly captivated by the qualities that set these influencers apart and made them the modern-day storytellers of their generation.

1. Authenticity in Aspiration: One of the first things that struck Kieran was the authenticity that underpinned the aspirations of these digital idols. They didn't just present a glossy facade of perfection; they shared their real-life journeys, complete with struggles, setbacks, and triumphs. It was as if they were inviting their followers to be part of their personal growth stories. Kieran admired how these influencers had the courage to be vulnerable, to open up about their insecurities and fears, and to show that the path to success

was filled with ups and downs. It was a refreshing departure from the unrealistic ideals often perpetuated in traditional media.

2. The Power of Storytelling: Kieran marveled at the way digital influencers harnessed the power of storytelling to captivate their audience. Each post was a carefully crafted narrative, a glimpse into their lives that left followers eagerly awaiting the next chapter. Whether it was a heartfelt story of overcoming adversity or a tale of an unforgettable adventure, these influencers knew how to evoke emotions and connect with their audience on a deeply personal level. Kieran aspired to be a storyteller like them, to weave narratives that resonated with people's hearts and souls.

3. Creating a Sense of Connection: What Kieran admired most was the sense of connection these influencers fostered with their followers. It wasn't just about amassing a large following; it was about building a genuine community of like-minded individuals who shared common interests and aspirations. Kieran saw how these influencers engaged with their followers, responding to comments, asking questions, and making their audience feel valued and heard. It was a sense of belonging that

Kieran longed for, a digital family where he could be his authentic self without judgment.

4. Empowerment Through Positivity: Kieran found inspiration in the way these digital influencers used their platforms to spread positivity and empowerment. Their messages were uplifting, encouraging their followers to chase their dreams, embrace their uniqueness, and overcome life's challenges. It was as if they had tapped into a wellspring of motivation and were sharing it generously with the world. Kieran wanted to be a source of empowerment, a beacon of hope for those who followed him, and he admired how these influencers used their influence for the greater good.

5. Curated Aesthetics: Beyond their personalities, Kieran was also enamored by the curated aesthetics of these influencers' profiles. The color schemes, visual consistency, and meticulous attention to detail created a sense of visual harmony that was pleasing to the eye. It was an art form in itself, and Kieran saw how it enhanced the overall appeal of their profiles. He learned that aesthetics were not just about vanity but a form of creative expression, a way to engage the audience on a sensory level.

6. Living Life to the Fullest: Perhaps what Kieran admired most was the way these influencers seemed to live life to the fullest. They embraced every moment with enthusiasm and a sense of adventure, turning even the most mundane activities into opportunities for discovery. Whether it was exploring a new city, trying exotic cuisines, or embarking on daring outdoor adventures, these influencers showcased a zest for life that was contagious. Kieran was inspired to seize the day, to embark on his own adventures, and to savor every experience with the same fervor.

As Kieran continued to explore the world of digital influencers, he realized that there was much more to admire beyond the polished images and curated personas. It was the authenticity, storytelling, sense of connection, empowerment, aesthetics, and zest for life that truly set them apart. These qualities were not just reserved for the digital elite; they were values and attributes that anyone could embrace and cultivate.

Amid the admiration he felt for digital influencers, there was a complex tapestry of emotions woven into Kieran's mental state. As he scrolled through their posts, he couldn't help but be aware of the stark contrast between the idealized lives they presented and the challenges he faced in his own reality.

At times, his admiration swelled into a sense of yearning, a deep longing to escape the confines of his ordinary life and step into the enchanting world these influencers inhabited. He would find himself daydreaming about the exotic destinations they explored, the glamorous events they attended, and the carefree adventures they embarked upon. It was as if he were living vicariously through their posts, seeking refuge from the mundane aspects of his daily existence.

Yet, intertwined with this yearning was a subtle undercurrent of insecurity. The flawless images and curated narratives of these influencers often left Kieran feeling inadequate and self-conscious. He couldn't help but compare his own life to the seemingly perfect worlds presented on his screen. The more he admired these digital sorcerers, the more he began to doubt himself and question his own worthiness.

This internal struggle with self-doubt cast a shadow on his mental state. Kieran grappled with a sense of inadequacy that gnawed at him from within. He wondered if he would ever measure up to the unattainable standards set by his idols. It was a battle that played out in his mind, a constant loop of comparison and self-criticism that eroded his self-esteem.

Additionally, the relentless pursuit of perfection that he observed among these influencers took a toll on his mental state. He felt the pressure to maintain a flawless online persona, to curate a life that mirrored the enchanting worlds of his idols. The quest for the perfect photograph, the most captivating caption, and the carefully constructed narrative became a source of anxiety and stress. Kieran was walking a tightrope between reality and illusion, and it was increasingly challenging to maintain his balance.

Yet, despite the turmoil in his mental state, Kieran couldn't deny the allure of these influencers. Their ability to transport him to a world of inspiration and aspiration was a lifeline in moments of self-doubt and insecurity. Their posts served as a source of motivation, encouraging him to chase his dreams and embrace the possibilities of life. It was a delicate dance between admiration and vulnerability, a tightrope walk that would define his journey in the world of "Digital Sirens."

As time passed, Kieran found himself increasingly consumed by the digital sirens of social media. The allure of these influencers had taken a firm grip on his psyche, and the lines between admiration and obsession had begun to blur. The perfection they portrayed, both in appearance and lifestyle, had become an unattainable ideal that loomed over him like a relentless shadow.

One of the aspects that weighed heavily on Kieran's mind was the pressure to look like these influencers. He couldn't escape the constant barrage of images showcasing impeccable skin, flawless physiques, and carefully curated outfits. As he admired their photos, he couldn't help but scrutinize his own reflection in the mirror, finding fault in every imperfection.

The acne scars that adorned his face, a reminder of battles fought and won, seemed like glaring flaws in comparison to the porcelain-smooth skin of his idols. He would spend hours researching skincare routines, trying out various products, and following regimens that promised to transform his complexion. The pursuit of the perfect skin, like that of his digital role models, became an obsession that left him feeling inadequate and self-conscious.

Kieran's physique, while in good shape, began to fall short of the sculpted bodies that were a hallmark of the influencers he admired. He started spending more time at the gym, pushing himself to the limits in pursuit of a chiseled physique. The pressure to conform to the standards of physical perfection set by his idols became a relentless force that drove him to extremes.

It wasn't just about physical appearance; it was also about the curated aesthetics of his photos. Kieran found himself constantly chasing the flawless lighting, the perfect angles, and the ideal settings that would mirror the polished images he admired. He became meticulous in his photo editing, using filters and retouching techniques to erase any perceived imperfections.

The pressure to look like these influencers was not just external; it had become an internal battle that waged within Kieran's mind. The desire to emulate their flawless appearance was a constant source of stress and self-doubt. He felt as though he were in a never-ending race, chasing an unattainable standard that left him perpetually dissatisfied with his own reflection.

The mounting pressure to look like his digital idols was taking a toll on Kieran's mental and emotional well-being. He grappled with a sense of inadequacy and self-esteem issues that seemed to intensify with each scroll through his social media feed. The pursuit of perfection had become an all-consuming endeavor that left little room for self-acceptance and self-love.

As the pressure to conform to the flawless standards set by his digital idols continued to mount, Kieran found himself hurtling down a treacherous path. The relentless pursuit of physical perfection was not without consequences, and it began to exact a toll on his mental and emotional well-being that extended far beyond his appearance.

One of the most noticeable changes was the increasing isolation from the real world. Kieran became so consumed by his quest to look like the influencers he admired that he withdrew from social interactions. Friends and family noticed his absence from gatherings and outings, and his once-vibrant social life began to wither away. The digital realm had become his primary focus, a place where he could escape into the illusion of perfection, leaving the real world behind.

He became increasingly detached from the people who cared about him, retreating into a self-imposed exile where he could obsessively edit photos, scrutinize his appearance, and curate his digital persona. Conversations with loved ones felt like distractions from his relentless pursuit, and he began to prioritize his online life over his real-life relationships.

The pressure to constantly improve his appearance became an all-consuming thought, occupying his mind to the point of obsession. It was as if he had been ensnared by a never-ending cycle of comparison, self-criticism, and the ceaseless pursuit of physical perfection. Each day brought a new set of anxieties about his looks, further isolating him from the joys and experiences of the real world.

Kieran's self-esteem continued to erode as he measured his self-worth solely by the unattainable standards of his digital idols. He felt a deep sense of inadequacy and self-doubt, plagued by the belief that he could never measure up to the flawless images he saw online. This toxic self-criticism became a constant companion, overshadowing any sense of self-acceptance or self-love.

Moreover, Kieran's preoccupation with his appearance began to affect his overall mental health. He experienced moments of anxiety and depression, triggered by the fear of falling short of the expectations he had set for himself. The relentless pressure he placed on his shoulders became a heavy burden that weighed him down, leaving him emotionally drained and mentally exhausted.

Days turned into weeks, and Kieran's isolation from the real world deepened. He missed out on important milestones in the lives of his friends and family, choosing instead to immerse himself in the digital realm where he could escape into the illusion of perfection. The moments of genuine human connection that had once brought him joy were replaced by the hollow validation of online likes and comments.

His sleep patterns became irregular, with late nights spent poring over photo editing apps and analyzing the profiles of his digital idols. The digital sirens of social media kept him awake, their voices urging him to strive for greater perfection, to never relent in the pursuit of the unattainable. The toll on his physical health was evident in the dark circles that formed under his eyes and the exhaustion that permeated his daily life.

As Kieran distanced himself from the real world, he began to experience a profound sense of loneliness. The digital realm, once a source of inspiration, had become a solitary confinement of his own making. He longed for genuine human connection, for conversations that went beyond captions and hashtags, for laughter that echoed in the real world, not just through the screens of his devices.

The more he isolated himself, the more his mental state deteriorated. He was trapped in a cycle of self-criticism, comparison, and anxiety, unable to break free from the prison of perfection he had constructed for himself. The real world, with all its imperfections and complexities, seemed distant and unfamiliar, like a place he could no longer access.

Kieran's preoccupation with his appearance reached a breaking point when he embarked on extreme measures to emulate the flawless physiques of his digital idols. He followed stringent diets, counted every calorie, and pushed himself to the limits at the gym. The pursuit of physical perfection had become an obsession that consumed his every waking moment.

His body, once a source of strength and vitality, had become a battleground in his quest for validation. He was driven to the brink of exhaustion by the relentless demands he placed on himself. The pressure to conform to the standards of his idols left him feeling physically drained and mentally overwhelmed.

Yet, no matter how much he pushed himself, no matter how closely he adhered to the regimens he had adopted, the idealized physique of his digital idols remained out of reach. The more he chased after their image of physical perfection, the further it seemed to recede into the horizon, a mirage that he could never quite grasp.

In his pursuit of the unattainable, Kieran's mental and emotional well-being continued to deteriorate. He became increasingly withdrawn, plagued by moments of self-doubt and despair. The disconnect between his online persona, "KaiZen," and his authentic self, Kieran, became a gaping chasm that seemed impossible to bridge.

The real-world consequences of his obsession with perfection were impossible to ignore. Kieran's relationships with loved ones had grown strained, his mental health was in a precarious state, and his physical well-being was suffering. He was on the precipice of a crisis, teetering on the edge of a precipice he had built with his own hands.

Chapter 3

The birth of ''Kaizen''

Little did Kieran know the profound transformation that "KaiZen" would undergo and the dark road that lay ahead. As he continued to cultivate his digital alter ego, the lines between his true self and his online persona began to blur in ways he could never have anticipated.

At first, the journey as "KaiZen" had been exhilarating. The followers poured in, and Kieran reveled in the attention and admiration. He basked in the sense of validation that came with each like and comment, each affirmation that he was indeed becoming the idealized figure he had aspired to be. The flawless world of digital social media seemed like a haven, a place where he could leave behind his insecurities and step into a world of unblemished perfection.

However, as "KaiZen" gained more and more followers, the pressure to maintain the facade intensified. The pursuit of perfection became an obsession, a relentless drive to outdo his previous posts, to maintain a consistent image of success and desirability. Kieran found himself spending hours each day curating content, editing images, and crafting captions that adhered to the persona of "KaiZen." It was a meticulous dance of pixels and words, a performance that left him emotionally drained.

The dark road that followed was one of isolation and anxiety. Kieran became increasingly disconnected from his real-life relationships as he poured more and more of himself into "KaiZen." He began to measure his self-worth solely in terms of his online presence, equating the number of followers and likes to his own value as a person. The relentless pursuit of perfection took a toll on his mental health, plunging him into a state of constant anxiety and self-doubt.

The pressure to maintain his digital alter ego became suffocating. Kieran felt trapped by the image he had created for himself, a prisoner of his own making. He was living a double life, juggling the demands of "KaiZen" with the realities of his authentic self. The dissonance between the two worlds became a source of inner turmoil, an emotional tug-of-war that left him feeling adrift and lost.

As he delved deeper into the digital realm, Kieran discovered the darker underbelly of social media. He encountered trolls and cyberbullies who attacked him with vicious comments and hurtful messages, eroding his self-esteem and fueling his anxiety. The relentless scrutiny and criticism from faceless strangers added to his growing sense of insecurity.

Kieran's descent into the abyss of his digital alter ego was a slow and insidious process. He had become addicted to the validation and affirmation that social media provided, and it had come at a steep cost. The very platform that had promised connection and inspiration had become a source of isolation and despair.

As the pressure to emulate his digital idols continued to consume Kieran, he found himself at a crossroads. The chasm between his real self and the digital personas he admired had grown so vast that it threatened to swallow him whole. He couldn't continue down this path of relentless self-criticism and isolation. It was time for a change, a transformation that would bridge the gap between the world he lived in and the digital dreamscape he aspired to join.

One evening, as Kieran sat alone in his dimly lit room, bathed in the eerie glow of his computer screen, inspiration struck. He had been scrolling through the profiles of his digital idols, once again comparing his own existence to the seemingly perfect lives they led. But this time, something clicked within him. It was as if a switch had been flipped, and a new idea began to take shape.

He pondered the concept of transformation, of becoming someone who could straddle both the real and digital worlds. What if he could create an alter ego, a digital persona that embodied the qualities and aspirations he admired in his idols? It would be an experiment, a way to explore the boundaries of identity and self-expression. Kieran felt a glimmer of excitement at the prospect of this audacious undertaking.

The name "KaiZen" flashed through his mind like a bolt of lightning. It was a fusion of two words: "Kai," representing change and transformation, and "Zen," symbolizing balance and harmony. It encapsulated his vision of a digital self that was in a constant state of improvement and growth, a persona that could inspire and uplift others just as his idols had inspired him.

With newfound determination, Kieran set out to create his alter digital self, "KaiZen." He started by meticulously planning his transformation, laying out a blueprint for the persona he wished to portray. It was an elaborate process that required careful consideration of every aspect of his digital identity.

1. The Visual Transformation: Kieran knew that the visual aspect would be key to crafting his digital persona. He began by revamping his wardrobe, selecting outfits that mirrored the fashionable ensembles of his idols. He invested in grooming products, skincare routines, and even experimented with makeup to conceal his acne scars. Each day, he practiced posing in front of the mirror, striving to capture the confident and carefree demeanor of his digital idols.

2. The Art of Storytelling: To create a compelling narrative for KaiZen, Kieran turned to the art of storytelling. He started by drafting a

list of experiences he wanted to have and adventures he wished to embark upon. These would become the backbone of his digital persona's story. He crafted captions and narratives that showcased KaiZen as a seeker of adventure, a fearless dreamer, and a relentless pursuer of personal growth.

3. The Online Aesthetics: Aesthetics played a crucial role in the presentation of KaiZen's digital identity. Kieran carefully selected filters, color schemes, and visual themes that would give his profile a cohesive and visually pleasing look. He paid attention to the layout of his posts, ensuring that they flowed seamlessly and created a harmonious visual experience for his followers.

4. The Art of Connection: Kieran recognized the importance of building a sense of connection with his followers, just as his idols had done. He began engaging with his audience more authentically, responding to comments, asking questions, and fostering a sense of community. He wanted KaiZen's followers to feel valued and heard, to experience a genuine connection that went beyond the surface of curated perfection.

5. Empowerment and Positivity: Central to KaiZen's persona was the message of empowerment and positivity. Kieran wanted his alter ego to inspire others to chase their dreams, embrace self-improvement, and overcome life's challenges. He crafted captions that carried messages of hope and motivation, encouraging his followers to believe in themselves and their limitless potential.

6. The Dual Existence: Maintaining the dual existence of Kieran and KaiZen was a delicate balancing act. Kieran decided that he would keep the two personas separate, revealing KaiZen only on his digital platforms. In the real world, he would continue to be Kieran, but online, he would transform into the embodiment of his digital dreamscape.

The creation of KaiZen was not just about emulation; it was an exploration of self-expression and self-discovery. Kieran viewed this alter ego as an experiment in identity, a way to explore the boundaries of authenticity and aspiration in the digital age.

The moment of truth came when Kieran posted his first image as KaiZen. It was a carefully crafted photograph taken during a trip to a picturesque mountain range. He stood on the edge of a cliff, arms outstretched, the wind tousling his hair. The backdrop of majestic peaks and a vibrant sunset created a breathtaking tableau. The caption read, "Embracing the beauty of the unknown. □ #AdventureAwaits #FearlessDreamer #Limitless."

The response was immediate and overwhelming. Likes and comments poured in, and within hours, KaiZen's following began to grow. It was as if he had unlocked a secret formula for digital enchantment, a way to transport his followers to a world of inspiration and aspiration.

The journey of Kieran and KaiZen had officially begun, and it was a path filled with both wonder and complexity. Kieran found himself navigating a dual existence, one foot in the real world and the other in the digital realm. Maintaining the balance between authenticity and aspiration would prove to be a challenging endeavor, and he was about to embark on a journey that would lead him deeper into the heart of "Digital Sirens."

With each post, each narrative, and each interaction, KaiZen began to take on a life of his own. He became a source of inspiration, a digital mentor who encouraged others to embrace self-improvement and personal growth. Kieran's experiment in self-transformation had yielded unexpected results, as KaiZen's influence extended beyond the digital realm.

Yet, even as KaiZen's digital presence flourished, Kieran couldn't shake the nagging feeling that he was living a dual existence. The disconnect between his real self and his digital alter ego weighed on him, leaving him questioning the authenticity of his online persona. He had ventured into uncharted territory, and the complexities of his journey were only beginning to unfold.

As the days turned into weeks and Kieran's alter ego, KaiZen, began to gain traction in the digital realm, he realized that maintaining the illusion of perfection required more than just a change in mindset. It demanded meticulous attention to detail and a willingness to refine every aspect of his digital identity.

One of the first steps in this refinement process was the art of photo editing. Kieran recognized that his idols' profiles were filled with flawless images that seemed to defy imperfections. To match this standard, he delved deep into the world of photo editing apps and software. Each photograph he took as KaiZen underwent a meticulous transformation.

With deft strokes of virtual brushes, he erased any blemishes or imperfections that marred his skin. The acne scars, which had once been a source of self-consciousness, were now mere memories, digitally concealed beneath a layer of retouching. Kieran became an expert at enhancing the clarity of his eyes, whitening his teeth, and sculpting his facial features with subtle adjustments.

But it wasn't just his complexion that underwent a digital makeover. Kieran experimented with filters, color grading, and lighting effects to infuse his photos with an ethereal quality. Each image was carefully curated to create an otherworldly atmosphere, as if KaiZen existed in a realm untouched by the imperfections of the real world.

The art of photo editing became an essential tool in maintaining the illusion of perfection, and Kieran's skills in this arena continued to evolve. It was as if he had become a digital magician, wielding the power to transform his appearance with the click of a button. The gap between his real self and his digital persona widened, and he found himself straddling the boundary between authenticity and artifice.

Beyond photo editing, Kieran began making subtle changes to his appearance in the real world. He adopted a meticulous skincare routine, investing in high-end products that promised to enhance his complexion. He experimented with hairstyles and grooming techniques to mimic the polished look of his idols. His wardrobe underwent a transformation, with an emphasis on fashion-forward attire that mirrored the stylish ensembles he admired in the digital elite.

The pursuit of perfection extended to his physique as well. Kieran intensified his fitness regimen, pushing himself to attain a physique that matched the sculpted bodies of his idols. He adhered to strict diets, monitored his calorie intake meticulously, and spent hours in the gym, sculpting his body into a work of art. Each muscle became a testament to his dedication, and he documented his fitness journey on his digital platforms.

As KaiZen continued to captivate his growing audience, Kieran's dual existence became more pronounced. The transformation of his appearance, both digitally and in the real world, seemed like a necessary sacrifice to maintain the illusion of perfection. It was a precarious balance between authenticity and aspiration, a tightrope walk that challenged his understanding of self.

In the digital realm, KaiZen's posts showcased a life of adventure, confidence, and effortless beauty. The curated aesthetics and flawlessly edited images painted a picture of a world untouched by imperfections. It was a world of endless possibility and boundless inspiration, a place where dreams came to life.

But as Kieran meticulously refined his digital identity, he couldn't help but wonder about the authenticity of it all. The real world, with its complexities, imperfections, and genuine moments, seemed increasingly distant. He had embarked on a journey of self-transformation, but it was a path fraught with contradictions, a journey that blurred the lines between self-expression and self-deception.

Kieran had always been drawn to stories of superheroes, individuals who possessed extraordinary abilities and could rise above any challenge. In the digital realm, KaiZen began to take on a similar role in Kieran's life—an embodiment of his ideal self, a digital superhero who shielded him from the complexities of reality.

As KaiZen's following continued to grow, Kieran couldn't help but see his digital persona as a superhero of his actual self. The transformation he had undergone was nothing short of remarkable, and KaiZen had become a symbol of his aspirations, a beacon of hope in the sometimes mundane world of Kieran.

In the real world, Kieran grappled with the challenges and imperfections of everyday life. He faced the pressures of work, the expectations of society, and the complexities of personal relationships. There were moments of self-doubt and uncertainty, moments when he felt vulnerable and imperfect.

But when he assumed the digital guise of KaiZen, it was as if he stepped into a different dimension—a world where he could transcend the limitations of his real self. KaiZen became the embodiment of confidence, courage, and resilience. He was a symbol of boundless potential, a digital hero who inspired others to overcome obstacles and chase their dreams.

KaiZen's posts were more than just carefully curated images and motivational captions; they were a source of empowerment and escape for Kieran. Each time he crafted a narrative, he felt a surge of confidence and determination. Each time he shared a story of personal growth, he was reminded of his own capacity for transformation.

The allure of this digital superhero was not lost on Kieran's growing legion of followers. They looked to KaiZen for inspiration and guidance, drawn to the charismatic persona that seemed to effortlessly navigate the challenges of life. It was as if KaiZen possessed an otherworldly wisdom, a superpower that could uplift and motivate those who followed his journey.

But as Kieran continued to embrace the role of KaiZen, he couldn't help but wonder about the impact of this dual existence on his connection with the real world. While KaiZen shielded him from the vulnerabilities of his real self, it also created a sense of dissonance. The gap between the digital superhero and the real Kieran grew wider, and he began to question the authenticity of his online persona.

The real world, with its complexities and imperfections, seemed increasingly distant. Kieran found himself spending more time in the digital realm, where he could escape into the illusion of perfection and inspiration. The pressures of reality paled in comparison to the allure of KaiZen's digital dreamscape.

It was as if Kieran had created a protective shield around himself, a shield that allowed him to navigate the challenges of life from a place of confidence and empowerment. But in doing so, he risked losing touch with the genuine moments of vulnerability and authenticity that defined the human experience.

As KaiZen continued to inspire and uplift others, Kieran grappled with the complexities of his dual existence. He was torn between the allure of the digital superhero and the need to reconcile his online persona with his real self. The journey of self-discovery he had embarked upon was leading him into uncharted territory, where reality and aspiration converged in a delicate dance.

As Kieran's journey in the digital realm continued, a subtle yet undeniable truth began to gnaw at the edges of his consciousness: KaiZen wasn't real. Despite the meticulous curation of images, narratives, and inspiration that he had poured into this digital alter ego, there was an essential hollowness to it all.

It was a realization that came to him one night, as he sat alone in the dim glow of his computer screen, scrolling through the profiles of his digital idols. He couldn't shake the feeling that there was something inherently artificial about the entire digital world he had created. The flawless images, the inspirational narratives, and the curated perfection—they were all masks, carefully constructed to shield him from the vulnerabilities of reality.

KaiZen, with his confident demeanor and boundless enthusiasm for life, had become a digital hero. But in that moment of self-reflection, Kieran couldn't help but see the stark contrast between his real self and this idealized persona. It was as if he had created a character, a larger-than-life figure, to navigate the digital world—a character that was not rooted in the authenticity of his true self.

The realization was both liberating and disconcerting. Liberating because it offered a glimpse of clarity—a recognition that the pursuit of perfection and inspiration in the digital realm had led him down a path of self-deception. Disconcerting because it meant acknowledging the distance between who he was and who he had portrayed himself to be.

Kieran struggled with the weight of this revelation. He had invested so much time, energy, and emotion into crafting KaiZen's identity that the line between reality and aspiration had blurred. He had become entangled in a web of his own creation, and the threads of authenticity were fraying.

For weeks, he grappled with conflicting emotions. He questioned the authenticity of his online persona and wondered if he had lost touch with the genuine moments of vulnerability and authenticity that defined the human experience. KaiZen, once a source of inspiration and empowerment, now felt like a mask that he could never fully remove.

Kieran's growing legion of followers, drawn to the charismatic persona of KaiZen, only deepened his internal struggle. They looked to him for guidance and inspiration, unaware of the complexities that lay beneath the surface. Kieran felt a sense of responsibility to these followers, a duty to continue being their digital mentor and motivator.

But the burden of maintaining this dual existence weighed heavily on him. He couldn't help but long for a sense of authenticity, a return to the genuine moments of connection and vulnerability that had defined his human experiences. The allure of the digital superhero had given way to a yearning for something more meaningful and real.

One evening, as he stared at his reflection in the mirror, Kieran made a decision. He knew he needed to confront the truth about KaiZen and come to terms with the complexities of his digital existence. It was time to let go of the illusion of perfection and embrace his true self, scars and imperfections included.

The process of dismantling KaiZen's digital identity was not easy. It required Kieran to step back from the digital world he had created and face the realities of his own imperfections. He began by sharing his struggles, his doubts, and his moments of vulnerability with his followers, dismantling the facade of unwavering confidence.

The response was both surprising and heartwarming. His followers, who had looked up to KaiZen as a symbol of inspiration, responded with empathy and understanding. They shared their own stories of imperfection and vulnerability, creating a sense of genuine connection that had eluded Kieran in his pursuit of perfection.

Kieran's journey was far from over, but it had taken a significant turn. He had come to terms with the complexities of his digital existence and had learned that authenticity, vulnerability, and imperfection were the true sources of human connection and growth. As he continued to navigate the digital world, he did so with a renewed sense of purpose and a commitment to being true to himself, scars and all.

Despite Kieran's initial resolve to let go of the digital alter ego, KaiZen, and embrace authenticity, he found himself unable to sever the ties completely. The allure of the digital superhero, with its veneer of perfection and boundless inspiration, continued to exert a powerful hold on him.

Kieran's internal struggle intensified as he grappled with the complexities of his dual existence. While he yearned for authenticity and genuine connection, he couldn't deny the seductive appeal of KaiZen's digital dreamscape. It was a world where he could escape the imperfections and vulnerabilities of reality, a world that offered him a sense of empowerment and invincibility.

In moments of self-doubt, Kieran found himself revisiting the carefully curated images and narratives that had defined KaiZen's digital identity. He wondered if there was a way to deepen the facade, to make KaiZen even more convincing. It was as if he had become addicted to the persona he had created, unable to let go of the illusion of perfection.

Kieran began to explore new depths of deception within the digital realm. He researched advanced photo editing techniques, seeking to refine his images even further. Filters and retouching tools became his allies, allowing him to sculpt his appearance to match the flawless personas of his digital idols. Acne scars disappeared, skin was smoothed to an ethereal perfection, and every photograph was a work of artistry.

But it wasn't just the visual aspects that Kieran sought to enhance. He delved into the world of storytelling, crafting narratives that painted KaiZen as an even more extraordinary figure. He invented thrilling adventures and tales of personal growth that seemed to transcend the bounds of reality. With each post, KaiZen became larger than life, a digital demigod who inspired awe and admiration.

Kieran's followers, unaware of the depths of his deception, responded with enthusiasm. The engagement on his posts soared to new heights, and his legion of admirers grew even more fervent. They saw KaiZen as a figure of unparalleled inspiration, a digital hero who could do no wrong.

But as Kieran continued to deepen the facade of KaiZen, he couldn't escape the nagging feeling that he was losing touch with his true self. He had ventured into a world of artifice and artistry, where the line between reality and aspiration had become blurred beyond recognition. The dual existence he had created was pulling him further away from the authenticity and vulnerability he had initially sought.

The real world, with its complexities and imperfections, seemed increasingly distant. Kieran found himself spending more time in the digital realm, where he could escape into the illusion of perfection and inspiration. The allure of the digital superhero had become an addiction, a never-ending quest to refine the facade and maintain the illusion of invincibility.

Kieran's struggle to let go and his obsession with deepening the facade of KaiZen had become a double-edged sword. While he yearned for authenticity and genuine connection, he was drawn deeper into the complexities of his dual existence. The pursuit of perfection had led him down a treacherous path, and he couldn't see a way out.

As Kieran delved deeper into the world of digital deception, he orchestrated a web of intricately woven falsehoods that masked his true identity with stunning precision. The divide between his real self and the digital persona, KaiZen, grew into a chasm of duplicity, and Kieran reveled in the art of deception.

KaiZen, with his charismatic charm and seemingly boundless positivity, was a character meticulously crafted to captivate his followers. To maintain this facade, Kieran devised a strategy that involved a careful blend of image manipulation, narrative construction, and the selective sharing of personal details.

One of the most potent tools in Kieran's arsenal was his mastery of photo editing. Every image posted as KaiZen underwent a meticulous transformation, erasing any trace of imperfection or vulnerability. Acne scars vanished into digital oblivion, wrinkles were smoothed into nonexistence, and blemishes were artfully concealed. The result was a flawless visage that seemed to defy the ravages of reality.

Kieran's followers marveled at the ethereal beauty of KaiZen, unaware that the image before them was a carefully constructed illusion. They aspired to emulate the perfection they saw in his photographs, believing that KaiZen was the epitome of self-improvement and personal growth.

But the deception didn't end with image manipulation. Kieran was equally adept at crafting narratives that painted KaiZen as a figure of unparalleled inspiration and achievement. He invented thrilling adventures and tales of personal growth, each designed to reinforce the image of KaiZen as a digital demigod.

In these narratives, KaiZen conquered mountains, traveled to exotic locales, and achieved remarkable feats of strength and endurance. His life seemed like an unending stream of excitement and achievement, a testament to the power of unyielding positivity and self-belief.

Kieran carefully curated the stories he shared, selecting details that painted KaiZen as a larger-than-life figure. He highlighted moments of triumph while omitting any hint of struggle or vulnerability. The result was a digital hero whose life appeared to be an unbroken string of victories.

As Kieran's followers immersed themselves in the world of KaiZen, they began to look to him for guidance and inspiration. His posts were filled with motivational quotes and affirmations, each carefully chosen to reinforce the image of KaiZen as a source of unwavering positivity and empowerment.

Kieran's selective sharing of personal details played a crucial role in the deception. He shared just enough about his life to create the illusion of authenticity but carefully omitted any details that might reveal his true identity. His followers felt a sense of connection with KaiZen, believing that they were glimpsing the real person behind the digital persona.

But the truth was far more complex. Kieran was living a dual existence, one foot in the real world as Kieran and the other in the digital realm as KaiZen. Maintaining the facade became a never-ending juggling act, a performance that demanded unwavering dedication to the art of deception.

As Kieran's following continued to grow, so did the pressure to maintain the illusion. He found himself trapped in a web of lies, unable to break free from the persona he had created. The more his followers looked up to KaiZen, the more Kieran felt compelled to continue the deception.

The duality of Kieran's existence began to take a toll on his mental and emotional well-being. He felt like an imposter, living a life that was increasingly disconnected from his true self. The authentic moments of vulnerability and imperfection that defined his human experience were buried beneath layers of deceit.

Kieran longed for the freedom to be himself, scars and all, but the allure of KaiZen's digital dreamscape was too strong to resist. He couldn't let go of the deception, fearing that it would shatter the illusion he had created and alienate his followers.

In the digital realm, KaiZen's posts continued to inspire and uplift, reinforcing the image of the flawless digital hero. His followers saw him as a source of boundless motivation, a mentor who could do no wrong. They looked to him for guidance in their own quests for self-improvement, unaware of the tangled web of lies that underpinned KaiZen's digital existence.

As the months passed, Kieran's deception became increasingly intricate. He fabricated friendships and interactions to bolster KaiZen's image as a charismatic and sociable figure. He even went as far as creating fake accounts to engage with himself, further blurring the lines between reality and fiction.

The pressure to maintain the facade grew with each passing day. Kieran was trapped in a digital web of his own making, unable to escape the persona he had created. The fear of losing his followers, of being exposed as a fraud, kept him ensnared in the deception.

During his school years, Kieran had faced a relentless battle with acne that left deep emotional scars alongside the physical ones. The relentless teasing and taunts from his classmates had etched painful memories into his psyche. It was during these trying times that Kieran had sought refuge in the world of KaiZen, using his digital alter ego as a shield against the cruelty of the real world.

The early years of high school had been particularly brutal for Kieran. His face bore the marks of acne scars, a visible reminder of the trials he had endured. The bullies, always quick to seize upon any perceived weakness, had honed in on his skin imperfections, using them as ammunition for their relentless attacks.

Kieran's daily routine was punctuated by the cruel remarks and hurtful gestures of his tormentors. They mocked his appearance, calling him names like "Pizza Face" and "Scar Boy." The laughter that followed each insult cut deeper than any physical pain.

He had tried various treatments and remedies, from prescription medications to over-the-counter creams, but the relentless acne refused to yield. Kieran's self-esteem plummeted as he withdrew into a shell of self-consciousness. His social interactions dwindled, and he began to avoid mirrors, unable to confront his own reflection.

It was in the midst of this dark period that Kieran stumbled upon the idea of KaiZen. As he scrolled through the profiles of his digital idols, he found himself drawn to their seemingly flawless appearances. These influencers appeared untouched by imperfections, their skin smooth and radiant, their lives an endless stream of adventures and triumphs.

In the depths of his despair, Kieran yearned to escape the harsh realities of his school life and become someone else, even if only in the digital realm. He began to experiment with photo editing apps, learning the art of concealing his acne scars and blemishes in images. The process offered a temporary reprieve, a fleeting glimpse of the flawless version of himself he aspired to be.

Kieran also started to craft narratives and captions that painted a picture of a confident and resilient figure. He shared stories of personal growth and self-acceptance, even as he struggled to embody these ideals in his everyday life. The act of crafting these narratives became a form of catharsis, a way to channel his pain into something positive.

As he honed his skills in image manipulation and narrative construction, Kieran realized that he could use this newfound expertise to create a digital alter ego—a persona that was everything he wished he could be. He gave this persona the name "KaiZen," a fusion of "Kai" representing change and "Zen" symbolizing balance.

KaiZen became an escape, a refuge from the relentless bullying he faced at school. When he logged into his digital platforms and assumed the role of KaiZen, he shed the insecurities and vulnerabilities that weighed him down in the real world. He became a digital hero, a source of inspiration and empowerment for others.

Kieran found solace in the positive feedback he received when he posted as KaiZen. His followers admired his seemingly boundless confidence and the captivating narratives of personal growth he shared. They looked to him for guidance and inspiration, completely unaware of the turmoil he faced outside the digital realm.

But KaiZen wasn't just a facade; he became a source of strength for Kieran in his daily battles against the bullies. When the taunts and insults became unbearable, Kieran would retreat into the persona of KaiZen, drawing upon the digital hero's unwavering positivity and resilience.

In those moments, he would remind himself of the stories he had crafted as KaiZen, tales of overcoming adversity and embracing one's imperfections. He would channel the confidence and courage of his digital alter ego, finding the strength to stand tall in the face of his tormentors.

Kieran's response to the bullies began to change. No longer did he cower in the face of their cruelty. Instead, he confronted them with a newfound sense of self-assuredness, using the lessons he had learned from his digital alter ego. He would respond with a calm demeanor and words of empathy, disarming his tormentors with a grace they couldn't comprehend.

It wasn't long before the dynamics began to shift. Kieran's newfound confidence and resilience drew the attention of his classmates, who began to question the motives of the bullies. Some even reached out to him privately, sharing their own struggles and insecurities.

In these moments, Kieran realized the power of the digital world to bring about positive change. KaiZen had not only served as a shield against the cruelty of the real world but had also empowered him to become a source of inspiration and support for others.

As Kieran continued to navigate the complexities of school life, the divide between his real self and his digital alter ego became more pronounced. KaiZen had served as a lifeline during a dark period of his life, but he knew that he couldn't continue to hide behind the facade forever.

In his early 20s, Kieran found himself entangled in a web of his own making. What had started as an escape from the relentless bullying in his school years had evolved into a complex dual existence that defined his life. Kieran, the real person behind the facade, had become increasingly dependent on KaiZen, the digital alter ego that shielded him from the complexities of reality.

The scars from his school years, both physical and emotional, still lingered. Acne had given way to acne scars, a permanent reminder of the pain he had endured. While the bullying had ceased, the insecurities it had bred remained deeply ingrained in his psyche.

Kieran had entered adulthood with a longing for acceptance and validation, a desire to be seen as more than the sum of his imperfections. He had graduated from school, found employment, and formed new friendships, but the wounds from his past continued to haunt him. The fear of rejection and judgment remained ever-present.

It was during this vulnerable period that Kieran sought refuge once again in the persona of KaiZen. He had become adept at maintaining the facade, refining his image manipulation skills and narrative construction techniques to perfection. The divide between his real self and his digital alter ego had grown wider, and Kieran felt increasingly compelled to hide behind the mask he had created.

KaiZen, with his charismatic charm and seemingly boundless positivity, had become Kieran's fortress against the uncertainties and insecurities of adulthood. When he logged into his digital platforms, he shed the weight of his imperfections and stepped into a world where he could be the hero of his own story.

The rituals of image manipulation became a daily routine. Kieran used filters, editing apps, and lighting effects to craft images that presented a flawless version of himself. The acne scars that marred his face disappeared, his skin took on an ethereal glow, and every photograph was a carefully orchestrated work of art.

The process offered a semblance of control over his appearance, a way to erase the perceived flaws that had haunted him for years. Kieran's followers marveled at the captivating images he shared as KaiZen, admiring the seemingly unattainable beauty he presented.

But it wasn't just about visual deception. Kieran had honed his storytelling skills to perfection. He created narratives that painted KaiZen as a figure of unwavering confidence and achievement. The stories of personal growth and triumph he shared were carefully curated to reinforce the image of a digital demigod.

Kieran found himself addicted to the positive feedback he received when he posted as KaiZen. His followers admired the seemingly boundless confidence and optimism of his digital alter ego, and they looked to him for guidance and inspiration. In their eyes, KaiZen was the embodiment of self-improvement and personal growth.

Yet, as Kieran reveled in the adulation of his followers, he couldn't escape the nagging feeling that he was living a lie. The real Kieran, with his vulnerabilities and imperfections, felt increasingly distant. He had become a master of deception, adept at concealing his true self behind the facade of KaiZen.

In his 20s, Kieran's reliance on KaiZen to navigate the complexities of adulthood deepened. The digital alter ego had become his shield against rejection and judgment. When he faced social situations or professional challenges, he would retreat into the persona of KaiZen, drawing upon the digital hero's unwavering confidence and positivity.

KaiZen became a crutch, a way for Kieran to cope with the anxieties and insecurities that plagued him. In the real world, he often struggled with self-doubt and a pervasive fear of inadequacy. But when he assumed the role of KaiZen, those insecurities seemed to evaporate, replaced by a sense of empowerment and invincibility.

In moments of self-doubt or anxiety, Kieran would remind himself of the narratives he had crafted as KaiZen, stories of overcoming adversity and embracing one's true potential. He would channel the charisma and resilience of his digital alter ego, finding the strength to face the challenges of adulthood with a sense of unwavering confidence.

The divide between Kieran's real self and his digital alter ego became increasingly blurred. He often found himself living a double life, one foot in the real world as Kieran and the other in the enchanting digital realm as KaiZen. Maintaining this delicate balance was a daily struggle, and Kieran couldn't help but wonder if he was losing touch with his true self.

KaiZen had served as a lifeline during his school years, helping him cope with the bullying and find a sense of empowerment. But in adulthood, the reliance on his digital alter ego had deepened, and the lines between reality and aspiration had become dangerously blurred.

Kieran's friends and acquaintances in the real world knew him as a confident and positive individual, mirroring the persona of KaiZen. They admired his unwavering optimism and the seemingly boundless self-assuredness he displayed. They had no reason to suspect the complexities that lay beneath the surface.

But the facade was taking its toll. Kieran's sense of self had become increasingly fractured. He longed for the freedom to be himself, to embrace his imperfections and vulnerabilities without fear of judgment. Yet, the allure of KaiZen's digital dreamscape was too powerful to resist.

As he navigated the challenges of adulthood, Kieran couldn't help but feel like an imposter. He knew that the perfection he presented as KaiZen was an illusion, a carefully constructed facade that concealed the insecurities and imperfections he couldn't bear to reveal.

Chapter 4
The Cafe

Sarah and Mark were Kieran's closest friends, and their bond was forged through years of shared experiences and unwavering support. They had been there for him through the ups and downs of life, and their friendship had become an anchor in the stormy seas of Kieran's existence.

Sarah was a vivacious and caring soul, known for her infectious laughter and boundless empathy. Her warm, hazel eyes seemed to see straight through the facades people wore, and she had an uncanny ability to make others feel heard and understood. She had a thriving career as a social worker, dedicating her life to helping others navigate their own challenges and adversities.

Mark, on the other hand, was the pragmatic and dependable force in their trio. With a keen sense of humor and an unshakable loyalty to his friends, he was the one they turned to in times of need. Mark had pursued a career in teaching, shaping young minds and instilling in them the values of kindness and resilience.

The three friends had met during their high school years, a time when they were all navigating the treacherous waters of adolescence. Kieran had been struggling with self-esteem issues and the emotional scars left by years of bullying. It was during this vulnerable period that Sarah and Mark had extended their hands in friendship.

Their first encounter had been unremarkable— a chance meeting in the school library. Kieran had been sitting alone, his head buried in a book, when Sarah and Mark had approached him with a friendly greeting. Sarah had noticed the isolation in Kieran's eyes and felt compelled to reach out.

"Hey, mind if we join you?" Mark had asked with a warm smile, pulling out a chair.

Kieran had been taken aback by their kindness. He had become accustomed to solitude, convinced that he was better off on his own. But something about Sarah and Mark's genuine warmth had melted his defenses.

That day marked the beginning of a lifelong friendship. Sarah, Mark, and Kieran had quickly become inseparable, spending their weekends exploring the nearby woods, sharing secrets, and supporting each other through the challenges of high school. They had laughed together, cried together, and faced life's uncertainties as a united front.

It was Sarah who had encouraged Kieran to open up about his struggles with self-esteem and bullying. She had listened attentively as he shared the pain of feeling like an outcast and the scars, both physical and emotional, that had haunted him. Sarah's compassionate nature had provided a safe space for Kieran to express his deepest fears and insecurities.

Mark, too, had been a pillar of strength during Kieran's darkest moments. He had stood up to bullies on more than one occasion, showing unwavering support for his friend. Mark's resilience and courage had been a source of inspiration for Kieran, a reminder that he didn't have to face his demons alone.

As they sat together in the cozy corner booth of their favorite café on that fateful day, their friendship had matured and deepened over the years. They were no longer the teenagers they had once been, but their connection remained as strong as ever.

The café, with its warm ambiance and the familiar scent of freshly brewed coffee, had become a sanctuary for their friendship. It was a place where they could retreat from the complexities of life and simply be themselves. In that café, they had shared countless conversations, dreams, and confidences.

Kieran had often sought solace in the company of Sarah and Mark during his most difficult moments. They had been there to lift him up when he was at his lowest, offering unwavering support and encouragement. The café had witnessed their laughter and tears, their shared triumphs and defeats.

On that particular day, as they settled into their familiar corner booth, the atmosphere was filled with a sense of anticipation. It had been a while since they had all caught up, and Kieran had something important to share. The café, with its cozy familiarity, seemed like the perfect setting for a conversation that would change the course of their lives.

As they began to talk and share stories of their recent experiences, the connection between them remained as strong as ever. The years had brought new challenges and adventures, but their friendship had remained a constant source of support and love.

Little did they know that the conversation they were about to have would lead to a revelation that would test the strength of their friendship and set Kieran on a path of self-discovery and authenticity. The café, with its comforting presence, would become the backdrop for a pivotal moment in their lives—a moment that would shape their journey together in ways they could never have imagined. Kieran had arranged to meet his two closest friends, Sarah and Mark, at their favorite café on a brisk Saturday afternoon. It had been a while since they had all caught up, and Kieran was looking forward to spending time with them. Yet, as he sat at a corner table, he couldn't help but feel a familiar unease settle in the pit of his stomach.

He glanced at his reflection in the café window, taking a moment to smooth his unruly hair and straighten his shirt. The image he saw was that of Kieran—the real Kieran, with the scars of his past etched into his face. The same scars he had spent years concealing behind the digital facade of KaiZen.

As Kieran waited for Sarah and Mark to arrive, he couldn't shake the nagging feeling that had plagued him for years. He had always been open and authentic with his closest friends, sharing his hopes, fears, and vulnerabilities. But when it came to KaiZen, he had maintained a wall of secrecy, guarding his digital alter ego like a closely held secret.

Sarah and Mark had been there for Kieran through thick and thin. They had witnessed his struggles with acne and the emotional scars left behind by years of bullying. They knew the depths of his insecurities and the moments of self-doubt that had defined his journey. Yet, he had never revealed the extent of his digital deception to them.

As Sarah and Mark entered the café, their warm smiles and enthusiastic greetings immediately put Kieran at ease. They were both aware of his struggles with self-esteem and had always been supportive. It was precisely this unwavering support that made the prospect of revealing the truth about KaiZen all the more daunting.

The conversation flowed effortlessly as they settled into their cozy corner booth. They shared stories of their recent experiences, laughed at inside jokes, and reminisced about their shared adventures. Kieran relished the genuine connection he had with Sarah and Mark—it was a world untouched by the complexities of his digital existence.

But as the conversation continued, Kieran couldn't help but feel the weight of his unspoken deceptions pressing down on him. He watched as Sarah animatedly described her recent promotion at work, her eyes glowing with excitement. Mark shared tales of his travel adventures, recounting the breathtaking landscapes he had explored.

Kieran was genuinely happy for his friends, but he couldn't help but compare their stories to the narratives he had crafted for KaiZen. While his friends spoke of real-life achievements and experiences, he had invented thrilling tales of conquests and triumphs for his digital alter ego. The divide between his two worlds had never felt wider.

As the conversation turned to social media, Sarah and Mark began sharing their own experiences with online platforms. They talked about reconnecting with old friends, sharing family updates, and the occasional political debate. Kieran listened intently, aware that he was about to navigate treacherous waters.

"So, Kieran," Sarah said with a playful grin, "you've been awfully quiet about your social media presence lately. Anything exciting happening in your digital world?"

Kieran's heart skipped a beat. He had anticipated this moment, the inevitable question about KaiZen's online persona. He hesitated for a moment, searching for the right words. But in that moment of hesitation, he felt the weight of his unspoken deceptions bearing down on him.

He considered deflecting the question, changing the topic, or offering a vague response. But Sarah and Mark were his closest friends, the ones who had been there for him through the darkest moments of his life. The thought of continuing to hide behind the mask of KaiZen in their presence weighed heavily on his conscience.

Taking a deep breath, Kieran decided to be honest. He owed it to his friends, and to himself, to reveal the truth about his digital alter ego. With a mixture of trepidation and determination, he began to speak.

"Actually, there's something I need to tell you both," Kieran said, his voice slightly trembling. "You know how I've always struggled with self-esteem, especially during high school?"

Sarah and Mark nodded, their expressions filled with empathy and understanding.

"Well," Kieran continued, "during those tough times, I created a persona on social media. I called him KaiZen. He's this confident, inspirational figure who seems to have it all together. I used him as a way to escape from the insecurities and imperfections I felt in real life."

He paused, searching their faces for a reaction. Sarah and Mark exchanged glances, their brows furrowed in concern.

"KaiZen's posts are all about positivity, personal growth, and inspiration," Kieran explained. "But the truth is, I've been crafting this persona to hide behind. The images I share are heavily edited, and the stories I tell are often exaggerated or entirely fictional."

There was a moment of silence as his friends processed this revelation. Then, Sarah reached out and gently placed her hand on Kieran's. "Kieran, we've always known that you've had your struggles, but we never expected you to carry such a heavy burden alone."

Mark chimed in, "We're your friends, and we're here to support you no matter what. You don't have to hide behind a digital persona to be accepted by us."

Kieran felt a wave of relief wash over him. Their understanding and acceptance were more meaningful than he could have imagined. He had been carrying the weight of his unspoken deceptions for so long, and now that he had shared his secret with his closest friends, it felt like a tremendous weight had been lifted from his shoulders.

As Kieran continued to explain his reasons for creating KaiZen, Sarah and Mark listened with empathy and compassion. They understood that his struggles with self-esteem and the scars of his past had led him down this path of digital deception. They reassured him that their friendship was built on trust and authenticity, not on the facade of a perfect persona.

Tears welled up in Kieran's eyes as he spoke about the pressure he had felt to maintain KaiZen's flawless image. He recounted the moments of self-doubt and the fear of being exposed as a fraud. He confessed that he had often yearned for the freedom to be himself, scars and all, without the burden of concealing his true identity.

Sarah and Mark offered words of comfort and encouragement. They reminded Kieran that his imperfections were what made him unique and real. They emphasized that they valued him for who he truly was, not for the digital persona he had created. Their unwavering support provided a sense of validation that Kieran had been yearning for.

"I've missed having real conversations with you," Kieran admitted, his voice filled with emotion. "I've been living this dual existence for so long that it's been hard to know where KaiZen ends, and I begin."

Mark nodded understandingly, "It's never too late to rediscover your true self, Kieran. We're here to help you navigate that journey, every step of the way."

Sarah added, "And you don't have to do it alone. Authenticity is a journey we can all take together."

With the weight of his secret finally shared, Kieran felt a renewed sense of hope. He realized that the support and understanding of his friends were the most valuable assets he could ever have. It was time to embrace his true self and let go of the digital facade that had imprisoned him for so long.

The trio continued their conversation, discussing their plans for the future and the adventures they hoped to embark on together. The atmosphere in the café had shifted, becoming one of warmth, acceptance, and genuine connection. Kieran felt like he was finally rejoining the real world, no longer burdened by the need to hide behind KaiZen.

As the hours passed, the sun dipped below the horizon, casting long shadows across the café. Kieran couldn't help but think about the path that lay ahead. He knew that the journey toward authenticity wouldn't be without its challenges, but he also knew that he had the support of true friends who would stand by him every step of the way.

The café, once a place of unspoken deceptions, had become a sanctuary of honesty and acceptance. Kieran realized that he no longer needed to seek refuge in the digital world to find validation. He had found it in the eyes of his friends and in the warmth of their embrace.

Before Kieran's transformation into a mental health advocate, he had been living a relatively quiet and unremarkable life. His struggles with self-esteem and the scars of his past were still very much a part of his daily existence, but he had not yet found a way to channel them into a meaningful purpose.

After the café meeting with Sarah and Mark, where he had shared his secret about KaiZen, Kieran felt a brief moment of relief and freedom. However, as time passed, he began to grapple with the consequences of his newfound authenticity.

The revelation about KaiZen had shaken his online persona, and he watched as some of his followers began to question the authenticity of his past posts. He received messages from individuals who felt betrayed, as if they had been deceived by his previous facade. Kieran was caught in a whirlwind of emotions, torn between the desire to be genuine and the fear of losing the support of his online community.

As the weeks turned into months, Kieran's online presence started to decline. The pressure to be authentic and maintain transparency weighed heavily on him. He felt like he was constantly under a microscope, with every post and interaction scrutinized for any signs of insincerity.

Offline, Kieran's relationships with Sarah and Mark also began to change. While they had initially been supportive of his decision to reveal his secret, the dynamics of their friendship shifted. Kieran couldn't help but feel like he was no longer the same person they had known for years. The carefree camaraderie they once shared seemed distant, replaced by a sense of unease and distance.

Kieran's own mental health began to deteriorate as he grappled with the consequences of his decision. He felt isolated and overwhelmed, unable to find a sense of belonging in either the digital or real world. The darkness that had haunted him in his school years returned with a vengeance, and he struggled to find a way out.

Sarah and Mark's unwavering support for Kieran during his battle with self-confidence was nothing short of extraordinary. In the days and weeks following the revealing café conversation, their friendship blossomed into an even deeper and more meaningful bond.

Sarah, with her natural empathy and understanding, became Kieran's confidante in ways he had never anticipated. She made it a point to check in on him regularly, whether through heartfelt text messages or spontaneous visits. She understood that Kieran's journey toward self-acceptance was not a linear path but a series of ups and downs.

One sunny afternoon, Sarah invited Kieran to join her for a leisurely walk in the park. As they strolled along the winding paths, the golden leaves crunching beneath their feet, Sarah listened intently as Kieran shared his innermost thoughts and fears.

"I still can't believe how accepting you and Mark have been," Kieran admitted, his voice tinged with gratitude. "I was so afraid that sharing my secret would push you away."

Sarah smiled warmly, her hazel eyes filled with reassurance. "Kieran, our friendship isn't built on secrets or facades. It's built on trust and authenticity. We've seen you at your best and your worst, and we've always stood by your side."

Over time, Sarah encouraged Kieran to be more open about his struggles with self-confidence, both online and offline. She gently reminded him that vulnerability was not a sign of weakness but a powerful tool for connection and growth. Together, they brainstormed ways to share his journey of self-acceptance with others who might be going through similar challenges.

Kieran took Sarah's advice to heart and began to write candid and heartfelt posts on his social media accounts. He shared his experiences of self-doubt, moments of triumph, and the importance of embracing imperfections. His followers responded with an outpouring of support and appreciation for his authenticity.

Meanwhile, Mark played a different but equally crucial role in Kieran's journey. He became

Kieran's accountability partner, helping him set realistic goals to boost his self-confidence. They embarked on a fitness journey together, attending gym sessions and outdoor activities. Mark's unwavering encouragement helped Kieran build both physical strength and self-esteem.

One memorable weekend, Mark invited Kieran to join a group hike to a nearby mountain. The challenging ascent was symbolic of the journey Kieran was on—a path filled with obstacles and steep inclines. With Mark's guidance and the camaraderie of their hiking companions, Kieran reached the summit, his chest heaving with exhaustion but his spirit soaring with accomplishment.

As they gazed out at the breathtaking panoramic view from the mountaintop, Mark clapped Kieran on the back and said, "You see, Kieran? Just like this hike, life has its ups and downs. But with determination and the support of friends, you can conquer any mountain, physical or emotional."

Kieran's transformation was gradual but profound. With Sarah's emotional support and

Mark's practical guidance, he started to rebuild his self-confidence one step at a time. He learned that it was okay to acknowledge his insecurities and that true strength came from facing them head-on.

Their friendship became a constant source of motivation for Kieran. Whenever he faced moments of self-doubt, he knew that he could turn to Sarah and Mark for encouragement. Their belief in his ability to overcome his insecurities became a beacon of hope on his journey toward self-acceptance.

Kieran's social media presence continued to evolve, reflecting his newfound authenticity. He shared not only his successes but also his setbacks, reminding his followers that self-confidence was a journey, not a destination. His vulnerability struck a chord with those who had followed his transformation, and he received messages from individuals who found inspiration in his story.

The café, where they had first shared Kieran's secret, remained a cherished meeting place for the three friends. It became a symbol of their enduring friendship and the safe haven where they could be their true selves. The café had witnessed their shared laughter, their tears, and their heartfelt conversations about life's challenges and triumphs.

As Kieran continued to embrace his true self, he realized that self-confidence was not about being perfect but about accepting his imperfections with grace and resilience. Sarah and Mark had played instrumental roles in helping him rediscover his self-worth and the power of authenticity.

Despite the unwavering support of Sarah and Mark, Kieran couldn't shake the looming presence of his alter ego, Kaizen. The weight of maintaining his digital persona continued to bear down on him, and he found himself caught in a web of new lies and deceptions.

As he became more involved in his advocacy work and expanded his presence on social media, the pressure to live up to the image of Kaizen intensified. He felt a constant need to project an image of success, confidence, and unwavering positivity, even when he was grappling with his own doubts and insecurities.

Kieran's followers had come to expect inspirational quotes, flawless photos, and uplifting stories from Kaizen. The persona he had created had taken on a life of its own, and Kieran felt trapped in the role he had crafted. He began to fabricate stories of personal triumphs and achievements to maintain the illusion of Kaizen's flawless existence.

One evening, Kieran found himself scrolling through his social media accounts, searching for the perfect image to post. He had spent hours trying to capture the ideal photograph, using filters and editing apps to enhance his appearance. His reflection in the mirror seemed to pale in comparison to the digital version of himself.

Sarah and Mark had noticed the toll this digital charade was taking on Kieran. They could see the exhaustion in his eyes, the way he constantly compared himself to the idealized version of Kaizen. They gently urged him to take a step back and prioritize his own well-being.

But the pressure to maintain the illusion of Kaizen was relentless. Kieran feared that if he let his guard down, his followers would abandon him, and the online world that had become his refuge would crumble. He convinced himself that he had to keep up the façade to continue making a difference in the lives of others.

As the lies continued to pile up, Kieran's internal struggle grew more pronounced. He felt like he was leading a double life—one as the confident and inspirational Kaizen and the other as the vulnerable and imperfect Kieran. The boundaries between the two personas blurred, and he began to lose sight of who he truly was.

One day, as Kieran sat alone in his apartment, he received a message from a follower who had been deeply moved by one of Kaizen's posts. The follower shared a personal struggle and expressed how Kaizen's words had provided a glimmer of hope in their darkest moments. Kieran's heart sank as he read the message, torn between the desire to help and the knowledge that Kaizen's inspiration was based on falsehoods.

Kieran knew that he had reached a critical crossroads in his journey. He had to make a choice—continue down the path of deception, or summon the courage to confront his digital alter ego and reveal the truth. The pressure of Kaizen had pushed him to the brink, and he could no longer ignore the toll it was taking on his mental and emotional well-being.

Chapter 5
Getting in to Deep

As the demands of Kaizen's online presence grew, Kieran felt an increasing need to keep up appearances. His followers had come to expect a certain level of opulence and success, and he believed he needed designer clothes, accessories, and trinkets to maintain that image. The pressure to showcase a glamorous lifestyle became overwhelming.

Kieran found himself scrolling through the Instagram profiles of successful influencers and celebrities, envy gnawing at him with each perfect photo. He saw their designer wardrobes, luxurious vacations, and expensive gadgets, and he believed that emulating their lifestyles would elevate Kaizen's image to new heights.

One evening, Kieran stumbled upon a high-end fashion brand that he believed would be the key to boosting Kaizen's appeal. The sleek suits, stylish accessories, and flashy jewelry seemed like the perfect fit for his digital alter ego. Without hesitation, he made his way to the brand's website and began adding items to his cart.

The total cost of his shopping spree was staggering. Kieran watched as the numbers on the screen ticked higher and higher. He knew he couldn't afford it, but the pressure to meet the expectations of Kaizen's followers pushed him to complete the purchase. He entered his credit card information, his heart racing as he confirmed the transaction.

The excitement of the purchase quickly faded as reality set in. Kieran realized that he had just maxed out his credit card on designer clothes and accessories that he couldn't afford. Panic washed over him as he contemplated the consequences of his impulsive decision.

Over the next few weeks, Kieran's financial situation spiraled out of control. He continued to make extravagant purchases, convinced that each new item would solidify Kaizen's image of success. He borrowed money from friends and family, inventing stories about urgent expenses and unexpected bills.

Sarah and Mark, who had always been a source of support, began to sense that something was amiss. They noticed Kieran's extravagant spending and the mounting debt that he seemed reluctant to discuss. Concerned for their friend's well-being, they confronted him about his financial struggles.

Kieran felt cornered, trapped between the desire to maintain Kaizen's image and the guilt of deceiving his closest friends. He lied to Sarah and Mark, fabricating stories about financial emergencies and unexpected expenses. He assured them that he had everything under control, even as his debts continued to grow.

As Kieran's financial situation deteriorated, he found himself in a web of lies and desperation. He borrowed money from acquaintances, promising to pay them back as soon as possible.

He took out loans with high interest rates to cover his mounting debts, all in a desperate attempt to maintain the illusion of Kaizen's opulent lifestyle.

The pressure of his financial burden weighed heavily on Kieran, both online and offline. He felt like a fraud, living a lie that was spiraling out of control. The pursuit of perfection on social media had led him into a dark and treacherous place, where the lines between reality and deception blurred.

The temptation of maintaining the appearance of Kaizen's lavish lifestyle proved too strong for Kieran to resist. As he returned some of the items he had purchased, he secretly clung to others, unable to part with the allure of designer clothes and accessories. The impulse to project an image of success on social media still gnawed at him.

Kieran's resolve weakened further when he encountered a new wave of influencer collaborations and sponsored content opportunities. Brands were eager to partner with him, offering free products and lucrative deals in exchange for posts that showcased their products. The allure of these opportunities, coupled with the promise of free designer items, was too enticing to ignore.

Without the knowledge of Sarah and Mark, Kieran accepted these brand partnerships and began accumulating even more material possessions. He justified his actions by convincing himself that these partnerships would help him recover financially and maintain Kaizen's image of success.

However, the financial burden of maintaining an extravagant lifestyle soon caught up with Kieran. He found himself trapped in a cycle of reckless spending and mounting debt once again. The weight of his financial mistakes bore down on him, leaving him in a state of despair.

Kieran's friends began to notice the return of his erratic behavior, and they sensed that something was amiss. They grew increasingly concerned about his well-being and questioned the sudden influx of new items and luxury possessions.

One evening, as Kieran struggled to keep up with the mounting bills, he received a phone call from a collections agency, demanding payment for a delinquent loan. Panic washed over him as he realized the gravity of his situation. The disastrous turn his spending had taken had pushed him to the brink of financial ruin.

Amid the mounting financial struggles and the disastrous turn his spending had taken, Kieran found himself making a decision that would push the boundaries of his deception even further. In a desperate attempt to maintain the illusion of a lavish lifestyle, he decided to pretend to buy a Porsche.

The idea had been planted in his mind when he came across a Porsche dealership during one of his escapades through the city. The gleaming sports cars on display seemed like the embodiment of success, and Kieran couldn't resist the allure. He knew he couldn't afford such a luxury purchase, but he also knew that a Porsche would make for an impressive addition to Kaizen's online persona.

Kieran entered the dealership, his heart pounding with a mix of excitement and guilt. He pretended to be a serious buyer, asking detailed questions about the various models and inquiring about financing options. The sales representative, unaware of Kieran's true financial situation, was eager to assist him in making what seemed like a high-stakes purchase.

Kieran test-drove a Porsche, relishing in the feeling of power and prestige that came with it. He snapped photos of himself behind the wheel, capturing the moment for his social media followers. The illusion of success was intoxicating, and Kieran convinced himself that this charade was necessary to maintain Kaizen's image.

But as he sat down with the sales representative to discuss financing and finalize the deal, a wave of guilt washed over him. The weight of his deception bore down on his shoulders, and he knew that he was treading on dangerous ground. The Porsche was an expensive luxury he couldn't afford, and pretending to make such a purchase would only dig him deeper into a financial hole.

In that pivotal moment, Kieran made a choice. He decided to step back from the brink of another disastrous financial decision. With a heavy heart and a sense of shame, he explained to the sales representative that he needed more time to consider the purchase and left the dealership, empty-handed.

As he walked away from the Porsche dealership, Kieran knew that he had narrowly escaped another trap of his own making. The allure of material possessions and the pressure to maintain an extravagant image had nearly pushed him over the edge. He realized that the path to authenticity and financial responsibility required him to confront the consequences of his actions and make choices that aligned with his true values.

Kieran's quest to maintain the illusion of wealth and luxury had led him to an elaborate charade—one that took him to some of the most upscale stores in the city. He had become adept at pretending to be a potential buyer, trying on high-end clothing and accessories, all in the pursuit of obtaining photos for his social media posts.

One day, he found himself in the prestigious watch section of Selfridges, a renowned department store that showcased a dazzling array of luxury timepieces. The gleaming glass cases held watches with price tags that seemed astronomical, but Kieran was undeterred. He believed that these watches would be the perfect addition to Kaizen's image.

Kieran approached one of the sales associates with an air of confidence, trying to mask the anxiety that churned in his stomach. He inquired about the watches on display, asking to see some of the most exclusive models. The sales associate, well-versed in catering to discerning clientele, eagerly complied.

As the sales associate presented the watches, Kieran marveled at their craftsmanship and elegance. He tried on one after another, each time posing in front of a mirror, capturing images of himself with the coveted timepieces. He knew that these photos would be a goldmine for his social media content.

The sales associate, unaware of Kieran's true intentions, offered detailed information about each watch, explaining their unique features and the craftsmanship behind them. Kieran nodded and asked probing questions, doing his best to maintain the facade of a serious buyer.

As he admired his reflection in the mirror, Kieran couldn't help but feel a sense of emptiness. The watches he tried on were symbols of wealth and status, but they held no real meaning for him. He wasn't interested in their intricate mechanisms or the prestige they represented. He was simply using them as props for his digital persona.

After spending what felt like an eternity in the watch section, Kieran finally thanked the sales associate and left the store, his phone filled with photos of himself wearing expensive timepieces. He couldn't shake the feeling of hollowness that had settled in his chest. The pursuit of an idealized image on social media had led him to forsake his own values and authenticity.

As he scrolled through the photos later that evening, Kieran's guilt grew. He had once again sacrificed his integrity to maintain Kaizen's image, and he couldn't deny the toll it was taking on his mental and emotional well-being. The facade he had created was becoming increasingly difficult to sustain, and he knew that he was on a path of self-destruction.

Kieran's desperation to maintain Kaizen's image of opulence and success had driven him to increasingly reckless measures. As he continued to accumulate expensive designer props and accessories for his social media posts, he found himself drowning in debt. To fuel his extravagant lifestyle, he resorted to taking out multiple credit cards, each one pushing him deeper into financial turmoil.

The allure of designer clothing, luxury watches, and high-end accessories had become an obsession for Kieran. He believed that these props were the key to maintaining Kaizen's image and retaining his online following. The pressure to showcase a life of glamour and extravagance weighed heavily on him, and he was willing to do whatever it took to keep up appearances.

One by one, Kieran applied for credit cards, often using falsified information to secure approval. He masked his mounting debts from existing cards, creating a tangled web of financial obligations that he struggled to keep track of. The credit limits on these new cards provided him with a temporary sense of relief, but he knew it was a precarious solution.

With each new credit card, Kieran's sense of financial responsibility eroded further. He used them to finance extravagant shopping sprees, buying designer clothes, luxury accessories, and props for his social media posts. The euphoria of each purchase was short-lived, replaced by the gnawing anxiety of mounting debt.

Kieran's friends, Sarah and Mark, began to notice the changes in his behavior. They observed his extravagant spending and the signs of financial distress that he couldn't conceal. Concerned for their friend's well-being, they confronted him about his reckless behavior.

"Kieran, we've noticed that your spending has spiraled out of control," Sarah said, her voice filled with worry. "It's clear that you're struggling financially, and we're here to support you through this."

Kieran hesitated, torn between the guilt of his deception and the fear of losing his friends' support. He knew that he had placed himself in an unsustainable financial situation, but the pressure to maintain Kaizen's image had clouded his judgment.

"I… I've been trying to keep up with the image I've created for Kaizen," Kieran confessed, his voice trembling. "I've taken out multiple credit cards to finance these purchases, and now I'm buried in debt."

Mark's expression softened with understanding. "Kieran, you don't have to face this alone. We're here to help you navigate this challenging situation and find a way out of it."

With the support of his friends, Kieran began to confront the financial disaster he had created. They helped him assess his debts and develop a plan to manage them responsibly. It was a daunting task, and Kieran felt the weight of his past decisions bearing down on him.

He started to cut back on his extravagant spending, making a conscious effort to live within his means. The credit cards that had once provided him with a sense of freedom were now a source of stress and anxiety. Kieran realized that he needed to address his debts systematically, focusing on paying them off one by one.

The journey toward financial recovery was arduous, and Kieran faced many challenges along the way. He had to come to terms with the consequences of his reckless spending and the deceit that had led him down this path. It was a humbling experience, one that forced him to reevaluate his priorities and confront the damaging effects of his obsession with maintaining an illusion of success.

The burden of mounting debt and the weight of his financial struggles took a disastrous toll on Kieran's mental health. As he grappled with the consequences of his reckless spending and the deception that had led him into this crisis, his emotional well-being began to unravel.

Kieran found himself plagued by anxiety and sleepless nights. The constant worry about his debts and the fear of exposure gnawed at him relentlessly. He would lie awake in the darkness, his mind racing with thoughts of impending financial ruin. The pressure to maintain Kaizen's image, even as he faced the grim reality of his financial situation, left him feeling trapped and suffocated.

Every new credit card statement that arrived in the mail was a reminder of his past mistakes, a haunting presence that seemed to mock him. The interest rates on his cards were exorbitant, and the minimum payments were a constant source of stress. He felt as though he was drowning in a sea of financial obligations, with no lifeline in sight.

Kieran's once-confident demeanor began to crumble. He became withdrawn and irritable, snapping at friends and family over minor disagreements. The shame and guilt of his deception festered within him, eating away at his self-esteem and self-worth. He felt like a fraud, living a double life that was unraveling at the seams.

The pressure to maintain Kaizen's image only intensified as his mental health deteriorated. He believed that he had no choice but to continue the facade, to project an image of success and opulence even as his world was crumbling around him. The disconnect between the digital persona he had created and the reality of his life weighed on him like an anchor, dragging him deeper into despair.

Kieran's friends, Sarah and Mark, watched with growing concern as their once-vibrant and confident friend spiraled into a dark abyss. They recognized the toll that his financial struggles and the pressure to maintain Kaizen's image were taking on his mental health. They knew that something needed to change, and they were determined to help him find a way out of this crisis.

One evening, as Kieran sat alone in his dimly lit apartment, the weight of his deception and the relentless pressure of his online persona became too much to bear. Tears welled up in his eyes, and a profound sense of hopelessness washed over him. He realized that he had reached a breaking point, and he couldn't continue down this destructive path.

In a moment of vulnerability, Kieran reached out to Sarah and Mark, pouring out his struggles and fears. He admitted that he was trapped in a cycle of deception and financial ruin, and that it was taking a devastating toll on his mental health. He felt as though he was on the verge of a breakdown, and he needed their support more than ever.

His friends listened with empathy, their hearts heavy with concern. They assured Kieran that he wasn't alone in this battle and that they would stand by him every step of the way. They encouraged him to seek professional help to address his mental health and to develop a plan for managing his debts responsibly.

With their support, Kieran began to take the necessary steps to prioritize his mental well-being. He sought therapy to address the anxiety and depression that had consumed him. It was a challenging process, but he was determined to confront the emotional scars left by his past mistakes.

Chapter 6
Tightrope

Kieran's life had reached a devastating low point. He was drowning in debt, his mental health was deteriorating, and his friends, Sarah and Mark, had grown increasingly frustrated with his lies and deception. The pressure to maintain Kaizen's image on social media had brought him to the brink of collapse.

His financial situation had become unmanageable. The credit card bills had piled up to staggering heights, and Kieran found himself unable to make even the minimum payments. The interest rates were devouring what little income he had left, leaving him with a sense of hopelessness and despair.

Kieran's mental health had also hit rock bottom. The relentless pressure to project an image of success and opulence had taken a toll on his self-esteem and self-worth. He struggled with anxiety and depression, often spending days holed up in his apartment, unable to face the world.

His friends, Sarah and Mark, had stood by him through thick and thin, but their patience was wearing thin. They had watched as Kieran continued to deceive not only his followers but also the people who cared about him the most. They had tried to offer support and guidance, but Kieran's stubborn determination to maintain his online persona had driven a wedge between them.

One evening, as Kieran sat alone in his dimly lit apartment, he received a text message from Sarah. It was a message that he had been dreading, a message that would force him to confront the consequences of his actions.

"Kieran, we need to talk," the message read. "It's time to face the truth."

Kieran's heart sank as he read those words. He knew that his friends had reached a breaking point, and he couldn't blame them. He had pushed them away with his lies and deception, and now he was about to face the consequences.

The meeting with Sarah and Mark was tense and emotional. They confronted Kieran about his reckless spending, his accumulating debt, and the toll that his online persona had taken on his mental health. Their frustration and concern poured out as they spoke.

"Kieran, we've been trying to help you for so long," Sarah said, her voice filled with sadness.

"But you've continued down this destructive path, and it's tearing us apart."

Mark added, "We can't stand by and watch you self-destruct any longer. You need to face the truth about what you've done and take responsibility for your actions."

Kieran felt a deep sense of shame and guilt as he listened to his friends' words. He had let them down, and he knew it. The weight of his deception and the consequences of his actions were crushing him, and he felt as though he had hit rock bottom.

The conversation with Sarah and Mark ended with a painful ultimatum. They told Kieran that they couldn't continue to support him unless he was willing to change. They urged him to seek professional help for his mental health, to develop a realistic plan for managing his debt, and to confront the truth about his online persona, Kaizen.

Alone in his apartment after the meeting, Kieran was overwhelmed with despair. He realized that he had pushed away the people who cared about him the most, and he was left to face the harsh reality of his situation on his own. The pressure to maintain Kaizen's image had led him to this point, and he had no one to blame but himself.

As the days turned into weeks, Kieran found himself in a deep abyss of despair. The ultimatum from his friends had left him feeling utterly isolated. He knew he had pushed them away with his lies and deception, and now he faced the daunting task of rebuilding their trust.

Kieran's mental health continued to deteriorate. The burden of his financial struggles, the weight of his past mistakes, and the isolation he felt all contributed to a growing sense of hopelessness. He struggled to get out of bed in the morning, and even the simplest tasks felt insurmountable.

The pressure to maintain Kaizen's image on social media remained relentless. Kieran found himself in a constant battle between the facade he had created and the truth he knew he needed to face. The allure of the online world, with its validation and likes, was a powerful force that seemed impossible to resist.

One evening, as he scrolled through his social media feed, Kieran came across a post from an influencer he had long admired. The influencer was living the kind of glamorous life that Kieran had always aspired to, with luxurious vacations, designer outfits, and an endless stream of adoring followers.

The post sent Kieran spiraling into a dark place. He compared himself to the influencer and felt an overwhelming sense of inadequacy. He believed that he would never measure up to the flawless images and lavish lifestyle that were portrayed online.

In that moment, the pain became too much to bear. Kieran felt as though he had hit rock bottom, and he saw no way out of the darkness that consumed him. The thought of ending it all seemed like the only escape from the suffocating pressure and the overwhelming despair.

But in the depths of his darkest moment, Kieran's phone rang. It was Sarah, calling to check on him. She had sensed his despair and knew that he was struggling. Her timing could not have been more critical.

Kieran hesitated for a moment, torn between the depths of his despair and the lifeline that Sarah represented. Ultimately, he answered the call, his voice trembling with emotion as he opened up to his friend about the pain he was feeling.

Sarah listened with compassion and empathy, her heart aching for her friend's suffering. She reminded Kieran that he was not alone in this battle and that there were people who cared about him deeply. She urged him to seek professional help immediately and assured him that he could overcome this darkness.

With Sarah's support, Kieran made a crucial decision to reach out to a mental health professional. He knew that he couldn't continue to battle his inner demons alone. The journey to healing would be long and challenging, but he was determined to confront the pain and despair that had brought him to the brink of self-destruction.

In the days that followed, Kieran's sense of despair seemed to deepen with each passing moment. He couldn't escape the overwhelming feeling that he had hit rock bottom, and the darkness that enveloped him felt all-consuming.

Every morning, he would wake up with a heavy heart, dreading the day ahead. The weight of his mounting debts and the guilt over the deception he had perpetuated pressed down on him like a suffocating blanket. The simple act of getting out of bed felt like an insurmountable task.

His apartment, once a place of refuge, had transformed into a prison of his own making. The walls seemed to close in on him, and the silence was deafening. Kieran felt utterly isolated, unable to reach out to his friends for fear of burdening them further.

The pressure to maintain Kaizen's image on social media continued to torment him. Every time he picked up his phone and logged into his accounts, he was bombarded with images of seemingly perfect lives and people who had it all together. He couldn't help but compare himself to these curated versions of reality, and he always came up short.

The online world, once a source of validation and connection, had become a source of torment. Kieran felt like an imposter, a fraud who had deceived his followers and lost touch with his true self. The dissonance between the image he projected and the reality of his life was tearing him apart.

One evening, as he sat alone in the dimly lit room, Kieran's thoughts took a dark turn. He felt as though there was no way out of the abyss he had fallen into. The weight of his past mistakes, the isolation he felt, and the relentless pressure to maintain an online persona became too much to bear.

In a moment of profound despair, Kieran began to entertain thoughts of ending it all. The idea of escaping the pain and the suffocating pressure seemed like the only way to find relief. He pictured a world where the torment would finally come to an end.

But as he contemplated this dark path, a small voice within him whispered that there might still be hope. It was a voice that remembered the love and support of his friends, Sarah and Mark, and the lifeline they had offered when he had needed it most. It was a voice that recognized the possibility of healing and redemption, even in the darkest of moments.

With great effort, Kieran pushed back against the thoughts that threatened to consume him. He reached out to Sarah once more, this time letting her know the depth of his despair. He confessed the darkness that had overtaken him and the thoughts that had plagued his mind.

Sarah responded immediately, her concern and care evident in her words. She reminded Kieran that he was not alone and that they would face this darkness together. She encouraged him to seek professional help, assuring him that there was a path to healing and recovery.

With Sarah's support, Kieran took the first steps toward confronting his mental health crisis. He reached out to a therapist and began the difficult process of untangling the emotional scars that had brought him to this precipice of despair.

Chapter 7
Healing

Kieran knew that he had reached a critical juncture in his life. The darkness of despair and the weight of his past mistakes had brought him to the edge of self-destruction. He couldn't continue to battle his inner demons alone, and he recognized that seeking professional help was the only way to navigate the treacherous path to healing.

With the support of Sarah, who had been his unwavering lifeline throughout this tumultuous journey, Kieran began the process of finding a therapist who could help him confront the emotional scars that had led him to this point.

The search for a therapist was both daunting and liberating. It marked the first step toward acknowledging the depth of his struggles and his commitment to recovery. Kieran was determined to confront the pain, guilt, and shame that had haunted him for so long.

After careful research and consideration, Kieran scheduled his first therapy session. It was a nerve-wracking experience, walking into a stranger's office and baring his soul. He feared judgment and condemnation, but he also longed for the chance to unburden himself of the emotional baggage that had become too heavy to bear.

The therapist, Dr. Amanda Turner, welcomed Kieran with warmth and empathy. Her office was a sanctuary of sorts, a safe space where Kieran could finally release the emotions that had been trapped within him for so long.

In their sessions, Kieran began to unpack the layers of his past. He spoke of the immense pressure to maintain Kaizen's image, the reckless spending, and the web of deception he had woven. He delved into the guilt he felt for pushing away his friends, especially Sarah and Mark, who had stood by him when he needed them most.

Dr. Turner guided Kieran through the process of understanding the root causes of his behaviors and the underlying emotional wounds that had driven him to create an alter ego online. It was a painful journey, filled with tears and moments of intense introspection, but it was also a path toward healing and self-discovery.

With each therapy session, Kieran began to gain insight into the patterns of behavior that had led him to this point. He realized that the pressure to maintain an image of success and perfection had been a way to compensate for feelings of inadequacy and low self-esteem. The online persona of Kaizen had become a shield, protecting him from the vulnerabilities and insecurities he had buried deep within.

Dr. Turner introduced Kieran to coping strategies and techniques to manage his anxiety and depression. She helped him develop a healthier relationship with social media, teaching him to distinguish between the curated online world and the reality of his life. Kieran learned to set boundaries, to focus on self-care, and to challenge the unrealistic standards he had imposed on himself.

As the weeks turned into months, Kieran's progress was slow but steady. The weight of his past began to lift, and he started to rebuild the shattered pieces of his self-esteem. He also reconnected with his friends, Sarah and Mark, who welcomed him back with open arms. They had seen the change in him, the newfound determination to confront his demons and embrace authenticity.

Kieran continued his therapy sessions, using each one as an opportunity to peel back another layer of his emotional baggage. He realized that healing was not a linear journey but a series of ups and downs, breakthroughs and setbacks. It required patience, self-compassion, and a commitment to ongoing self-improvement.

As Kieran continued his therapy sessions with Dr. Turner, he began to notice subtle but significant shifts within himself. The healing process was gradual, but each breakthrough brought him closer to a place of self-acceptance and self-compassion.

One of the most transformative aspects of therapy for Kieran was the opportunity to confront his innermost feelings of guilt and shame. Dr. Turner encouraged him to explore the roots of these emotions and to challenge the unrealistic expectations he had placed on himself.

Kieran learned to forgive himself for the mistakes he had made in his pursuit of the online persona, Kaizen. He realized that he was not defined by his past actions but by his capacity for growth and change. This newfound sense of self-forgiveness allowed him to release the heavy burden of guilt that had haunted him for so long.

The therapy sessions also provided Kieran with tools to manage his anxiety and depression. He practiced mindfulness techniques that helped him stay grounded in the present moment, rather than getting lost in the idealized images of social media. Breathing exercises and meditation became part of his daily routine, providing a sense of calm and stability.

With Dr. Turner's guidance, Kieran began to rebuild his self-esteem from the ground up. He recognized the value of self-compassion and self-care, learning to prioritize his own well-being over the unrealistic standards he had imposed on himself. He started to see his worth beyond the number of likes and followers on social media.

Kieran's friends, Sarah and Mark, continued to stand by his side throughout this transformative journey. They had seen the profound changes within him and celebrated each milestone with him. Their unwavering support was a constant reminder that he was not alone in this battle.

One day, Kieran decided to face the truth about Kaizen head-on. He posted a heartfelt message on his social media accounts, acknowledging the deception he had perpetuated and the pain it had caused him and others. He explained that he was on a path to self-discovery and authenticity and that he would no longer strive to maintain a false image of perfection.

The response from his followers was mixed. Some applauded his honesty and vulnerability, while others criticized him for breaking the illusion they had admired. But Kieran no longer sought validation from the online world. He had found a sense of self-worth and authenticity that was far more valuable than the fleeting approval of strangers.

As Kieran's journey of self-acceptance and authenticity unfolded, he encountered a series of moments that continued to shape his evolution.

One of those pivotal moments occurred when he decided to share his story openly on a larger platform. He wrote a heartfelt blog post detailing his experiences, the allure of social media perfection, and the toll it had taken on his mental health. The post resonated with many, as it touched on the universal struggle to reconcile the curated online world with the complexities of real life.

Kieran's blog post garnered significant attention and support from readers who had faced similar challenges. They shared their own stories of striving for digital perfection and the subsequent impact on their well-being. The sense of community and understanding that emerged from these interactions reinforced Kieran's commitment to living authentically and using his experiences to help others.

Kieran's newfound passion for photography flourished as he embraced authenticity in his work. He began capturing raw, unfiltered moments that celebrated imperfections and vulnerabilities. His photos conveyed a sense of honesty and emotion that resonated with viewers far more profoundly than the polished images he had once strived to create.

One of the most powerful changes in Kieran's life was his ability to cultivate self-compassion. He learned to be kind to himself, recognizing that everyone makes mistakes and faces struggles. Self-criticism gradually gave way to self-love and acceptance, allowing Kieran to embrace his true self with a newfound sense of confidence.

Throughout this journey, Kieran remained connected to his therapist, Dr. Turner. Their sessions shifted from introspection to practical strategies for navigating the complexities of modern life. Together, they explored topics like setting healthy boundaries with social media, managing stress, and fostering resilience.

Kieran's relationship with Sarah and Mark continued to thrive. Their bond grew deeper as they embarked on adventures that celebrated authenticity and connection. Kieran had come to value their friendship not for the number of likes or followers it brought but for the genuine support and understanding they shared.

Kieran's work in volunteering and giving back to the community became an integral part of his life. He found fulfillment in making a positive impact on the lives of others, proving that authenticity could extend beyond the self and into the world around him.

Though Kieran's journey had been transformative, he knew that it was a continuous process. The allure of social media's perfection and the pressures of the digital age would always be present, but he had developed the inner strength to navigate them with authenticity.

As Kieran's journey of self-acceptance and authenticity continued, he found himself on a path of ongoing growth and self-discovery.

One significant aspect of his transformation was his evolving perspective on success and happiness. Kieran had once equated success with the pursuit of external validation and material possessions. Now, he understood that true success was rooted in personal fulfillment, meaningful relationships, and a sense of purpose.

He began to prioritize his well-being above all else, recognizing that mental and emotional health were the cornerstones of a fulfilling life. Kieran continued to attend therapy sessions with Dr. Turner, using them as a tool for self-reflection and personal growth.

Kieran's photography became a reflection of his journey toward authenticity. He captured moments that celebrated the beauty of imperfection and the richness of genuine human connections. His work resonated with an audience eager to embrace the authenticity he portrayed, and he found a growing community of like-minded individuals who valued vulnerability and realness.

In his blog and social media posts, Kieran shared not only the highlights of his life but also the challenges and setbacks. He wanted his online presence to be a place where others could find inspiration and solace in the knowledge that they were not alone in their struggles.

Kieran's commitment to giving back to the community grew stronger. He volunteered regularly, using his experiences to inspire and uplift others. His work became a testament to the power of authenticity in making a positive impact on the world.

One of the most profound changes in Kieran's life was his ability to form deep and meaningful connections with others. His friendships with Sarah and Mark continued to thrive, and he welcomed new people into his life who shared his values and passions. Kieran had learned that authenticity not only attracted authentic people but also allowed him to forge genuine connections.

Despite the ongoing challenges and temptations of the digital age, Kieran remained resolute in his commitment to living authentically. He understood that the journey was a continuous one, filled with moments of self-reflection and growth. He was no longer afraid to confront his vulnerabilities and imperfections, for he had come to see them as a source of strength and authenticity.

As Kieran's journey of authenticity continued to unfold, he encountered both challenges and triumphs, each contributing to his growth and self-discovery.

One of the challenges he faced was the occasional pull of old habits and the allure of the digital persona he had once created. There were moments when the pressure to conform to societal standards of perfection tempted him to return to his former ways. However, Kieran had developed a strong sense of self-awareness and resilience that allowed him to resist these temptations.

Kieran's blog and social media presence became a platform for discussions on authenticity, mental health, and the pitfalls of pursuing digital perfection. He shared not only his own experiences but also the stories of others who had embarked on similar journeys toward self-acceptance. His audience continued to grow, and his words resonated with those seeking a more genuine and meaningful connection in the digital age.

In his personal life, Kieran continued to nurture his friendships with Sarah and Mark. Their bond had deepened, and they celebrated each other's successes and supported one another through life's challenges. Kieran had learned the true value of authentic friendships and the importance of surrounding oneself with people who embraced imperfections.

Kieran's photography evolved to reflect his journey. He captured moments of vulnerability, joy, and authenticity, using his art to convey the beauty of being true to oneself. His work gained recognition not for its polished aesthetics but for the emotions it conveyed.

Throughout this ongoing process, Kieran remained committed to giving back to the community. His volunteer work became a source of fulfillment and purpose, and he continued to make a positive impact on the lives of others.

One of the most significant triumphs in Kieran's life was the realization that authenticity was not a destination but a lifelong journey. He understood that self-acceptance and embracing imperfections required constant self-reflection and growth. Kieran had come to appreciate the beauty of living in the present moment, free from the constraints of a curated digital persona.

As Kieran's story continued to unfold, he faced new challenges and celebrated new victories in his quest for authenticity. The road ahead was filled with opportunities for growth, self-discovery, and a deeper understanding of what it meant to live a truly authentic life in a world dominated by the allure of digital perfection.

One of the most profound transformations in Kieran's life was his redefinition of success. He no longer measured success solely by external achievements or the approval of others. Instead, he found success in the small, meaningful moments that brought him joy and fulfillment.

Kieran continued to prioritize his mental and emotional well-being. Therapy with Dr. Turner remained an essential part of his life, offering him a safe space for self-reflection and personal growth. He understood that ongoing self-awareness was key to maintaining his authenticity in a world that often encouraged conformity.

His photography continued to evolve as well. Kieran's work became a powerful form of self-expression, capturing the beauty of everyday life, imperfections and all. He used his art to convey the depth of human emotions and the essence of authenticity, resonating with those who valued the genuine over the staged.

Kieran's blog and social media presence continued to inspire others to embrace their true selves. He shared not only his triumphs but also his moments of vulnerability and self-doubt, showing that authenticity was a journey that required courage and self-compassion.

His friendships with Sarah and Mark remained steadfast. Together, they celebrated their authentic selves and the unique qualities that made each of them special. Kieran had come to understand that true friendships were built on acceptance and genuine connection, not on the pursuit of perfection.

Kieran's commitment to giving back to the community grew stronger. He found ways to make a positive impact on the lives of others, using his experiences and his platform to advocate for mental health awareness and the importance of embracing authenticity.

Throughout his ongoing journey, Kieran realized that authenticity was not a destination but a way of life. It was a commitment to being true to oneself, even in the face of societal pressures and the allure of digital perfection. He knew that the road ahead would continue to present challenges, but he faced them with resilience and a deep sense of purpose.

As Kieran's story continued to unfold, it served as a beacon of hope and inspiration for others seeking to live authentically in a world that often valued conformity. His journey was a testament to the power of self-discovery, self-acceptance, and the enduring beauty of imperfection.

Chapter 8
Self Worth

Kieran's remarkable journey toward self-worth and authenticity, he stood at the pinnacle of personal transformation. His path had led him to a place where he not only cherished his self-worth but also inspired others to embark on their own quests for authenticity and self-acceptance.

The Blossoming of Self-Worth

Kieran's understanding of self-worth had evolved into a deep and unshakable sense of self-acceptance. He had transcended the need for external validation or social media metrics to affirm his value. Instead, he drew strength from within, recognizing that his worth as an individual was inherent and unchangeable.

Therapy with Dr. Turner had played a crucial role in Kieran's journey. Their sessions had shifted from exploring past wounds to focusing on practical strategies for maintaining a healthy sense of self-worth. Dr. Turner had helped Kieran dismantle the barriers of self-doubt and instilled in him the tools to navigate moments of insecurity.

Kieran's digital alter ego, Kaizen, had once served as a shield against vulnerability. Kieran now understood that it had been a manifestation of his own self-sabotage—a way to avoid confronting his inner insecurities. This realization had empowered him to face his vulnerabilities with courage and self-compassion.

Photography as a Canvas of Authenticity

Kieran's photography had undergone a remarkable transformation. No longer did he seek to enhance his images with filters or digital alterations. Instead, he aimed to capture the unfiltered beauty of life—the raw emotions, imperfections, and genuine connections. His photography had become a visual testament to the power of authenticity.

His work resonated deeply with an audience yearning for authentic human expression. People from all walks of life found solace and inspiration in Kieran's photos, which conveyed a sense of authenticity and raw beauty. His art served as a catalyst for others to embrace their true selves and find beauty in imperfections.

Inspiring Authenticity Through Online Presence

Kieran continued to use his blog and social media presence as a platform for inspiration and empowerment. His posts were not mere showcases of personal achievements but candid reflections of his struggles, vulnerabilities, and moments of self-doubt. His authenticity resonated with his followers, offering a relatable voice in an age dominated by curated perfection.

Through his posts, Kieran urged his audience to embark on their own journeys of self-discovery and self-worth. He believed that by sharing his experiences and insights, he could help others break free from the suffocating pressures of perfection and external validation. His words became a source of strength for those seeking to reclaim their authenticity.

The Resilience of Authentic Friendships

Kieran's friendships with Sarah and Mark had grown even more profound. Their bond was a testament to the enduring power of genuine connections. They celebrated each other's growth and authenticity, reinforcing the value of acceptance, empathy, and shared experiences in their lives.

These friendships had been pivotal in Kieran's journey. They served as a constant reminder that authentic connections thrived on acceptance and the appreciation of each other's imperfections. Kieran cherished the support system that had unwaveringly stood by him throughout his transformation.

Giving Back and Cultivating Self-Worth in Others

Kieran's commitment to giving back to the community had expanded further. He had taken on initiatives designed to nurture self-esteem and self-worth in others, particularly among young individuals. He believed that by helping them recognize their inherent value, he could contribute to a world that celebrated authenticity over superficiality.

Through workshops, talks, and community outreach, Kieran harnessed his experiences and platform to advocate for mental health awareness and the importance of self-acceptance. He inspired young minds to embrace their uniqueness and reject the unrealistic standards perpetuated by digital culture.

The Ongoing Journey

In this chapter of Kieran's life, he stood not only as a beacon of hope but also as a catalyst for change. His journey was a testament to the enduring power of healing, self-discovery, and the beauty of embracing one's true self, imperfections and all.

As Kieran's story continued to unfold, he understood that the road ahead was filled with opportunities for further growth, self-reflection, and the perpetual practice of authenticity. His life had become a living testament to the resilience of the human spirit and the transformative power of embracing one's true self in a world often consumed by illusions.

In Kieran's ongoing journey toward self-worth and authenticity, he had not only discovered the intrinsic value of his true self but also learned to navigate the digital landscape without falling into the traps of social media and the allure of influencers.

Guarding Against the Traps of Social Media

Kieran had developed a set of mindful practices to guard against the pitfalls of social media. He recognized that the curated perfection presented online could lead to feelings of inadequacy and self-doubt if not approached with care. To maintain his self-worth, he:

1. Limited Comparison: Kieran consciously avoided comparing himself to others on social media. He knew that curated images often did not reflect the reality behind the scenes, and he refused to measure his worth by these superficial standards.

2. Filtered His Feed: He curated his social media feed to include content that aligned with his values and promoted authenticity. He followed accounts that celebrated imperfections, mental health awareness, and genuine human connections.

3. Scheduled Digital Detoxes: Kieran regularly took breaks from social media to reconnect with the offline world. These digital detoxes allowed him to recenter himself and maintain a healthy perspective on the digital realm.

4. Practiced Mindfulness: Mindfulness meditation had become an integral part of Kieran's daily routine. It helped him stay grounded and present, reducing the anxiety and pressure often associated with social media.

Navigating the Influencer Culture

Kieran had also cultivated a critical mindset when it came to influencers and their impact on self-worth:

1. Authenticity Over Glamour: He reminded himself that the glamorous images presented by influencers were often the result of meticulous curation and editing. Kieran valued

authenticity over glamour and appreciated influencers who shared their real experiences.

2. Fostering Real Connections: Kieran focused on building genuine connections with people who shared his values rather than idolizing influencers. He understood that real relationships were far more valuable than superficial admiration.

3. Supporting Authentic Influencers: He actively supported influencers who used their platforms to promote authenticity, mental health awareness, and body positivity. Kieran believed in uplifting those who made a positive impact on the digital landscape.

4. Media Literacy: Kieran practiced media literacy by critically evaluating the content he consumed. He questioned the motives behind sponsored posts and scrutinized the authenticity of influencer endorsements.

The Ongoing Journey of Self-Worth and Authenticity

Kieran's journey toward self-worth and authenticity had reached a point of profound self-assuredness. He was no longer swayed by the facade of social media or the allure of influencers. Instead, he had learned to harness the digital realm as a tool for inspiration, connection, and empowerment.

His commitment to self-worth extended beyond his personal growth. Kieran continued to inspire and support others on their own journeys of authenticity. He used his online presence as a platform to advocate for a more genuine and compassionate digital culture, where self-worth was measured by inner strength and acceptance, not by external metrics.

As Kieran's story continued to evolve, he remained a beacon of hope and resilience for those who sought to navigate the complexities of self-worth and authenticity in a world often dominated by superficiality. His ongoing journey was a testament to the enduring power of self-discovery and self-acceptance, even in the face of digital illusions and external pressures.

Kieran's ongoing journey was a testament to the enduring power of self-discovery and self-acceptance in a digital age fraught with illusions and pressures. He stood as a guiding light, showing that authentic self-worth could flourish even in the face of social media's curated perfection.

Chapter 9
Breaking Free and Help

If you or someone you know is struggling with issues related to self-worth, authenticity, and the challenges associated with social media and digital personas, there are several avenues where help and support can be found:

1. Therapy and Counseling: Seeking the guidance of a mental health professional, such as a therapist or counselor, can be incredibly beneficial. They can provide a safe space to explore these issues, develop coping strategies, and work on building self-worth.

2. Support Groups: Many support groups, both online and offline, focus on self-esteem, self-worth, and related issues. Connecting with others who are facing similar challenges can provide a sense of community and shared understanding.

3. Mental Health Organizations: Organizations like the National Alliance on Mental Illness (NAMI), Mental Health America (MHA), and others offer resources, support, and information on mental health topics.

4. Online Communities: Online communities and forums dedicated to mental health, self-esteem, and self-acceptance can be valuable sources of support. However, it's essential to verify the credibility and safety of these platforms.

5. Self-Help Books and Resources: There are many self-help books and resources available that focus on building self-worth, authenticity, and navigating the challenges of the digital age. These can provide valuable insights and strategies.

6. Meditation and Mindfulness: Practicing mindfulness and meditation can help individuals become more grounded, reduce stress, and improve self-awareness. Many apps and online resources offer guided meditation sessions.

7. Seeking Professional Guidance: For those struggling with digital personas and the pressure to maintain a perfect online image, seeking guidance from a social media expert or

life coach can provide valuable insights into managing online presence and expectations.

It's important to remember that reaching out for help is a sign of strength, and there is no shame in seeking support when facing these challenges. If you or someone you know is in immediate crisis or experiencing thoughts of self-harm or suicide, please reach out to a crisis hotline or a mental health professional immediately. Your well-being is of utmost importance, and help is available.

8. Educational Workshops: Many organizations and mental health institutions offer workshops and seminars on topics related to self-esteem, digital well-being, and navigating social media. These can provide practical skills and insights.

9. University Counseling Centers: For students in college or university, counseling centers often offer free or low-cost counseling services to help address mental health concerns, including those related to self-worth and social media.

10. Apps and Online Tools: Several mental health apps and online tools are designed to

promote self-awareness, self-esteem, and digital well-being. Examples include mindfulness apps, self-help apps, and mood tracking tools.

11. Peer Support: Connecting with friends or peers who have experienced similar struggles can be a source of understanding and encouragement. Sharing experiences and strategies can be mutually beneficial.

12. Social Media Detox Programs: Some organizations and therapists offer structured social media detox programs designed to help individuals take a break from or reduce their social media usage. These programs can be effective in reducing the negative impact of social media on mental health.

13. Local Community Resources: Community centers, libraries, and local organizations may host support groups or workshops related to mental health and self-esteem. These can be excellent resources for finding local support.

14. Professional Life Coaching: Life coaches specialize in helping individuals set and achieve personal and professional goals. They can provide guidance on self-discovery and developing a sense of purpose.

15. Holistic Approaches: Exploring holistic practices like yoga, art therapy, or nature therapy can be beneficial for improving self-worth and finding inner balance.

16. Hotlines and Crisis Support: In moments of crisis or severe distress, hotlines such as the National Suicide Prevention Lifeline (1-800-273-TALK) or crisis text lines can provide immediate support.

The Samaritans helpline is an excellent resource for individuals who are experiencing emotional distress, crisis, or need someone to talk to. The Samaritans offer emotional support 24 hours a day, 7 days a week, and can be reached at different phone numbers depending on your location. Some of the main helpline numbers are:

- United States: National Suicide Prevention Lifeline at 1-800-273-TALK (1-800-273-8255)
- United Kingdom and Ireland: Samaritans at 116 123 (Freephone)
- Canada: Crisis Services Canada at 1-833-456-4566
- Australia: Lifeline Australia at 13 11 14

- New Zealand: Lifeline New Zealand at 0800 543 354
- India: Snehi at +91 22 2772 6770

These helplines provide confidential and non-judgmental support for individuals who may be experiencing emotional struggles, loneliness, crisis, or thoughts of self-harm or suicide. Trained volunteers are available to listen, provide emotional support, and offer guidance on seeking help.

If you or someone you know is in immediate danger or experiencing a crisis, please do not hesitate to reach out to the appropriate crisis hotline for your region. Your well-being is important, and there are compassionate individuals ready to help.

17. Family and Friends: Lean on trusted family members and friends for emotional support. Sometimes, talking openly with loved ones can be a significant first step in seeking help.

Remember that finding the right support system and resources may take time, and it's essential to seek help from qualified professionals when necessary. The journey to improved self-worth and authenticity is unique for each individual, and there are many avenues available to provide guidance, understanding, and assistance along the way.

18. Online Forums and Communities: There are various online communities and forums dedicated to mental health, self-esteem, and personal growth. Websites like Reddit have subreddits where individuals can share experiences and receive advice from peers.

19. Art and Creative Expression: Engaging in creative activities such as art, writing, music, or dance can be therapeutic and help individuals express their emotions and thoughts in a healthy way. Art therapy and creative expression workshops may be available locally.

20. Self-Compassion Practices: Learning and practicing self-compassion techniques can be transformative. Resources like books and online courses on self-compassion can help individuals develop greater self-acceptance.

21. Professional Life Coaching: Consider working with a certified life coach who specializes in personal development and self-

worth. They can provide guidance, motivation, and accountability on your journey.

22. Academic Courses: Some universities and educational institutions offer courses on topics like self-esteem, emotional intelligence, and well-being. These courses can provide valuable insights and skills.

23. Nature and Outdoor Activities: Spending time in nature and engaging in outdoor activities can have a positive impact on mental health. Nature therapy or ecotherapy involves using natural settings to support well-being.

24. Podcasts and Webinars: Many podcasts and webinars feature experts discussing topics related to self-worth, mental health, and personal growth. These can offer valuable insights and guidance.

25. Journaling: Keeping a journal to record thoughts, feelings, and experiences can be a therapeutic practice. Journaling can help individuals gain clarity, identify patterns, and track their personal growth.

26. Professional Social Media Consultation: If struggling with the pressures of social media and digital personas, consider consulting with a professional social media strategist or consultant

who can provide guidance on maintaining a healthy online presence.

27. Volunteer Work: Engaging in volunteer activities and helping others can boost self-esteem and provide a sense of purpose. It allows individuals to focus on making a positive impact in their communities.

28. Mindful Technology Use: Practicing mindful and intentional use of technology can help mitigate the negative effects of excessive screen time. Setting boundaries and screen-free times can promote digital well-being.

29. Books and Literature: There are numerous self-help books, memoirs, and literature that explore themes of self-worth, authenticity, and navigating the digital age. Reading such material can provide inspiration and guidance.

30. Emergency Helplines: In situations of crisis or immediate distress, don't hesitate to call emergency helplines, such as 911 (or the local equivalent), or reach out to a crisis hotline for immediate support.

It's essential to recognize that seeking help and support is a sign of strength and courage. Everyone's journey is unique, and there are a multitude of resources and strategies available to help individuals like Kieran overcome challenges related to self-worth and authenticity. The path to healing and growth may involve a combination of these resources and practices, and individuals should choose what resonates most with them on their journey.

31. Positive Affirmations: Incorporate positive affirmations into daily routines. Repeating affirmations that reinforce self-worth and self-acceptance can gradually change thought patterns.

32. Professional Development Workshops: Some workshops and seminars focus on personal development and building self-esteem. These can be valuable for gaining insights and practical skills.

33. Peer Mentoring: Connecting with a peer mentor who has overcome similar challenges can provide guidance, empathy, and motivation. Peer mentoring programs may be available in educational institutions or community organizations.

34. Online Courses: Consider enrolling in online courses that cover topics like self-worth, authenticity, and digital well-being. Many

reputable platforms offer courses on personal development.

35. Body Positivity Communities: If body image is a concern, explore body positivity communities and resources that encourage self-acceptance and challenge unrealistic beauty standards.

36. Financial Counseling: If financial pressures related to social media consumption are affecting well-being, seek financial counseling to address budgeting and debt management.

37. Mindful Social Media Usage: Practicing mindfulness while using social media involves being present and aware of emotional responses. Mindful techniques can help individuals navigate online spaces more healthily.

38. Art Therapy: Art therapists use creative processes to help individuals explore emotions and self-worth. Participating in art therapy sessions with a qualified therapist can be transformative.

39. Positive Role Models: Identify and follow positive role models online and offline—individuals who embody the values of authenticity and self-worth. Their stories and actions can be a source of inspiration.

40. Community Centers: Local community centers often host events, workshops, and support groups related to mental health and personal development. Check with community resources for offerings in your area.

41. Personal Growth Apps: There are apps designed to support personal growth and self-improvement. These apps offer various tools, exercises, and resources for building self-esteem.

42. Holistic Health Practices: Explore holistic approaches like yoga, meditation, acupuncture, or herbal therapy, which can promote mental and emotional well-being.

43. Continued Therapy: For individuals who have undergone therapy or counseling, it's essential to continue with maintenance sessions to ensure ongoing support and growth.

44. Community Volunteering: Engage in community service or volunteer work to build self-worth through contributing to the well-being of others.

45. Online Mental Health Resources: Websites and organizations dedicated to mental health, such as the National Institute of Mental Health (NIMH), provide extensive resources and information on various mental health topics.

46. Journal Prompts: Usc journaling prompts to delve deeper into self-reflection and self-discovery. Prompts can help individuals explore their feelings and thoughts.

47. Personalized Self-Care Plans: Create personalized self-care plans that include activities and practices that promote well-being and self-worth. Consistently implementing self-care routines can be transformative.

Remember that each individual's journey is unique, and it may involve a combination of these resources and strategies. Seeking help and support is a proactive step toward self-improvement and personal growth. It's essential to be patient with oneself and to recognize that self-worth and authenticity are ongoing pursuits that can evolve over time.